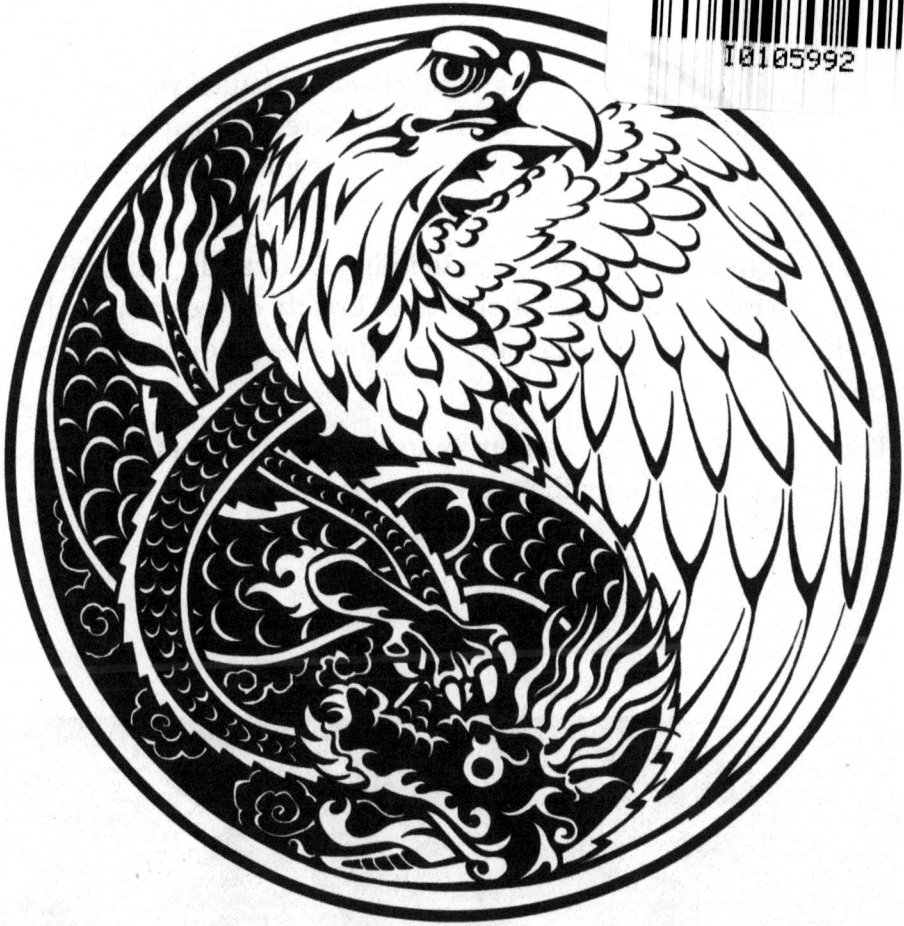

SAMMA

SEATTLE ASIAN MEDICINE AND MARTIAL ARTS

An Introduction to Tai Chi

SAMMA Tai Chi Student Manual

Disclaimer

Although the drills, exercises, and practices contained within this book are generally safe when performed correctly, instruction in tai chi is most appropriately obtained under the guidance of a qualified instructor.

Any exercise program can result in injury, and tai chi is no different. If you experience pain, shortness of breath, or feel faint or dizzy, discontinue your practice and consult with a medical professional.

The author assumes no responsibility or liability for injury sustained while performing the exercises in this book.

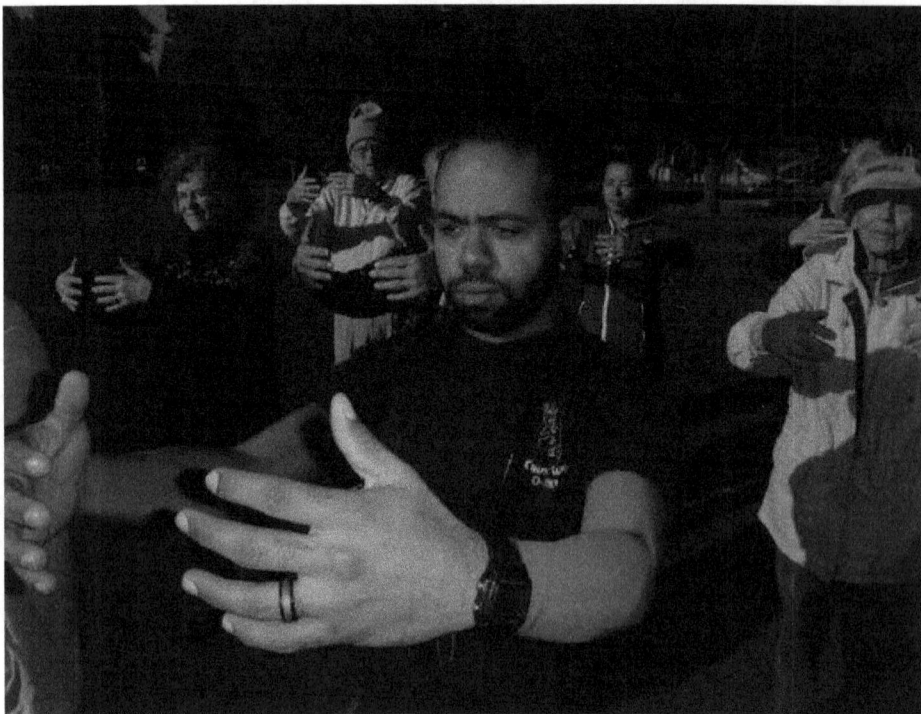

Foreword

The goal of this book is to provide students of tai chi with a road map to understand the theories and practices of this beautiful and sublime art. This book will be particularly helpful to the novice practitioner as it covers the majority of relevant introductory material. Supplemental materials are available that will explain some of the more advanced drills, forms, and weapons in detail.

My first exposure to tai chi was from my kung fu teacher Sifu Robert Brown in the 1980s. At this time, the slow and gentle movements did not make much sense to me. In 2004 I began the study of tai chi in earnest and I found my current tai chi teacher, Dr. Boonchai Apichai in 2005. Along the way, I have studied both Yang and Chen styles of tai chi, and have had many wonderful teachers to practice with, bounce ideas off of, and guide my understanding of this most difficult and elusive of arts. In spite of these efforts, mastery eludes me, and I hope only to get better over time.

From my perspective, I'm not convinced that mastery of tai chi is possible. Rather, we practice to simply improve our skill and depth of understanding. We peel off layers of tension and coarse, awkward body movements. We learn how to be more relaxed, breathe more deeply, move with confidence and ease, and find strength in an ever-deepening root to the ground beneath our feet. We find that we can access our true selves through the application of the principles of tai chi.

In your travels through tai chi be patient and focus on the journey and not the destination. In fact, I would argue that there is no destination in tai chi. There is only the process of discarding the static remnants of a life lived in survival mode to reveal a life that can thrive.

Note that tai chi originated in China. Because Chinese is a pictographic language, translation into English presents occasional challenges. It is common to find a variety of different English words to describe the same concept in tai chi, including the word tai chi itself, which is perhaps more accurately translated as "taiji". These different translations are based on different transliteration and translation systems used in academia. The two main systems are Pinyin and Wade-Giles, with Pinyin being the more modern version. I have used a mix of both in this manual, and I have tried to err on the side of what I believe is the most common usage of a word.

Additionally, it is possible to find the word "chuan" attached to the end of "tai chi". "Chuan" can be translated as "fist" and it often is used to denote a martial art. In the system I teach, I leave off the word "chuan" from our tai chi, as I do not teach the corresponding self-defense or martial arts applications. Although fighting applications are sometimes discussed in class because I have found that students are sometimes better able to conceptualize physical movements after seeing them applied in this context, this in no way substitutes for actual martial arts training.

Thank you to all of the teachers who pointed me in the right direction and all of the students who allowed me to explore.

Special thanks to Dr. Jeffrey Wong and Kay Uribe for graciously appearing as demonstrators in this book.

I take full responsibility for all errors, omissions, and mistakes found herein.

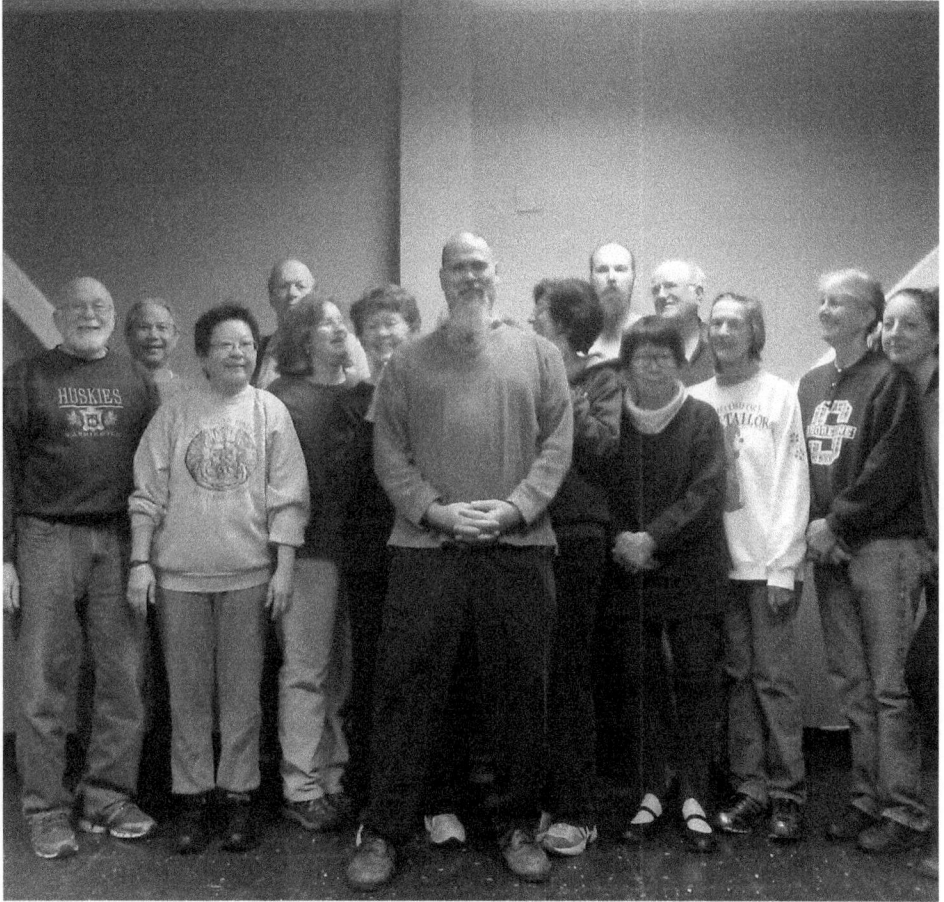

Tai Chi Students

Third Place Books, Seattle

2015

Table of Contents

Table of Contents

Table of Contents

Introduction

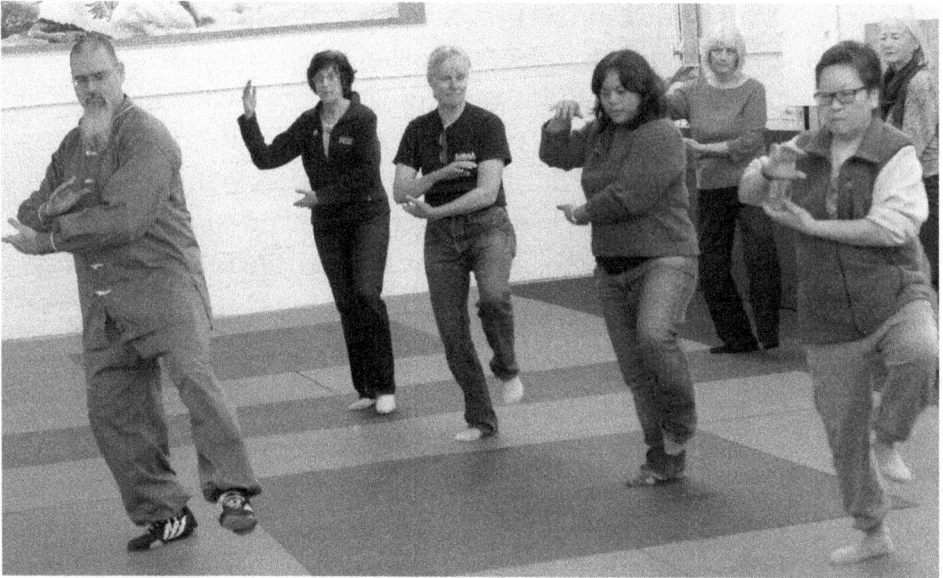

Tai Chi Performance at the SAMMA Grand Opening, 2013

This book is intended to help students develop a deeper appreciation for the art and science of tai chi. I have endeavored to include the theoretical concepts, warm-ups, exercises, drills, basics, and training methods necessary to develop proficiency in tai chi. A more detailed explanation of the individual forms, weapons, and push hands can be found in the author's other written materials.

What is tai chi?

Tai chi is a gentle and slow-moving exercise that safely and effectively improves health and well-being. It is a mind-body practice that originated in China hundreds of years ago that focuses on breathing and relaxation and is well known to reduce the harmful effects of stress. Although it is commonly known to improve fitness and balance in seniors, aid in relaxation, and improve health, it is less well-known that tai chi can be a meditative and spiritual practice, a system of self-defense, and a way to cultivate internal energy.

Sometimes students want to know the difference between tai chi and qi gong. Broadly speaking, tai chi is a specific set of practices, initially intended to be a martial art or self-defense. In the modern era, it is also commonly used for health improvement and stress reduction. Qi gong is any of a number of systems intended to work with your body's internal energy, which we call "*qi*". Sometimes, we characterize the difference as follows: tai chi is stillness inside and movement outside, qi gong is stillness outside and movement inside. Qi gong does not require any connection to tai chi; however, your tai chi practice should include one or more qi gong sets. Ultimately, the pursuit of either or both should have a positive impact on your life and your health.

The appendix includes a list of academic and physical competencies detailing the individual skills that make up the practice of tai chi. It is intended as a reference to be periodically checked against the student's progress.

Why study tai chi?

There are many reasons to study tai chi. Many scientific studies have demonstrated the positive impact on health – fall reduction in seniors, improvements to the quality of life in seniors with chronic health conditions, improved muscle strength, balance, and flexibility, reduced stress, lowered blood pressure, and many more. Other reasons include an improved sense of well-being and relaxation, self-defense, and disciplining the mind.

Tai chi is a deep well to draw from and will provide a lifetime of opportunities to learn and grow. There is no endpoint to the study of tai chi.

History

The origin of tai chi is lost to antiquity. It is commonly agreed that sometime in the 13th century, a man named Chang San-Feng practiced a martial art that mirrors what we have inherited as tai chi. One story suggests he was inspired to create a martial art system after observing a crane and a snake fight. Remnants of this story can still be seen in tai chi moves with names like "Snake Creeps Low" and "White Stork Spreads Wings".

At some point this art made its way to the Chen Village in Northen China where it was practiced and developed for centuries. All of the great tai chi schools trace their origins back to this village. A number of tai chi masters have gone on to found their own schools of tai chi.

Practicing Tai Chi

The road to mastery in tai chi is not an easy one to tread; progress is often measured by feet and not miles. The most important things to remember are to breathe and relax. Don't get frustrated if you can't remember exactly how to perform a movement or exercise, just practice as best as you can while remembering to breathe and relax.

There is no destination in tai chi, there is only the process of unwinding a lifetime of tension and cultivating your qi. There is no plateau that you will reach where you "know" tai chi. We strive for incremental improvements. In this journey, you will achieve the benefits that tai chi has to offer.

The following are some suggested ways to practice outside of class, to assist you on your journey.

1. **Horse stance.** Practice the small horse stance until your legs and back are strong enough to switch to the traditional horse stance. Start with 30 seconds, and try to increase the time that you can hold the stance each week. Focus on breathing deeply into your *tan tien*. Practice sinking your *qi* into the ground.

2. **Tai Chi Walking.** This exercise can be done anywhere, and it is one of the first skills a student will pick up. In addition to helping you master an important tai chi skill, it can be done to improve relaxation and concentration, practice integrating root and breath with movement, and help the student to differentiate *yin* and *yang*. Practice opening and closing your *kua*.

3. **Empty hand form.** Do whatever you can remember from the empty-hand forms, and practice them everyday. It's ok if it's not perfect. Make note of areas of the form that you are not sure about and ask in class for clarification. Once you have learned the sequence (and also while you are still learning) practice integrating the correct breath.

3. **Empty hand form.** Practice feeling for your root with each step. Pay attention to your structure—as you settle into each posture make sure that your hands and feet are in the correct position, that your eyes are looking in the correct direction, and that you are moving through your *tan tien*. It is particularly helpful to repetitiously practice the transitions from the form. Practice the form slowly (aim for about six minutes) but occasionally practice it fast.

4. **Tai Chi Qi Gong.** This is a great stand-alone warm-up sequence for your tai chi practice. It will reinforce the lessons from the empty-hand forms and improve health and fitness levels.

5. **Cultivate *qi*.** Broadly speaking, eating a healthy diet, getting high quality sleep, managing stress, and reducing destructive habits (alcohol, tobacco, drugs, etc.) are beneficial to your *qi*. Regular practice of energy cultivation exercises such as Minor Universal Circulation Qi Gong or Open Wisdom Qi Gong are enormously helpful, as are many other mindfulness practices.

6. **Warm-up exercises.** The stretches and warm-up exercises are intended to enhance your tai chi practice and improve your health. They are gentle enough on your body that they can be done for a few minutes every day. In particular, doing rotations daily will keep your joints healthy and facilitate the flow of *qi*.

7. **Relaxation techniques.** Practice any breathing and relaxation techniques you have learned, including qi gong, yoga, or meditation.

8. **Cultivate patience.** There are no shortcuts to the acquisition of skill. There is only practice. Through consistent practice, you will continue to improve.

Benefits of Tai Chi

There are many benefits to the practice of tai chi. These benefits are regularly confirmed through decades of scientific and medical studies and research, but more importantly, they are experienced in the daily lives of millions of students. Tai chi is a safe and effective weight-bearing (helps the bones) and cardiovascular exercise (helps the heart and lungs) that uses only the weight of your body. It requires no tools, no high-velocity changes in direction of motion, and no high impact or repetitive physical contact that may lead to injury.

When looked at through the lens of Traditional Chinese Medicine (TCM), tai chi is an exercise system that cultivates our body's vital internal energy without depleting it. This energy, which we call "*qi*", tends to get stagnant in our joints which in turn leads to diseases like arthritis. The postures in tai chi move the limbs, torso, and joints allowing the *qi* to flow more harmoniously and therefore prevent disease.

- **Improves strength and balance** (1). Tai chi has been found to reduce the risk of falls in seniors and has been shown to reduce the effects of osteoarthritis.

- **Reduces symptoms of Parkinson's disease** (2). The practice of tai chi had a positive effect on Parkinson's disease.

- **Improves strength** (3). Regular practice of tai chi improves muscular strength.

- **Gives a boost to cognitive function** (4). There is a growing body of evidence that suggests that tai chi practice can improve memory and cognitive abilities, particularly in seniors.

- **Improves COPD symptoms** (5). One study found that tai chi can help patients with COPD walk and exercise better, an another study found that tai chi helped boost exercise capacity and endurance in people with COPD.

- **Improves sleep** (6). A trial study found that tai chi improved sleep duration, sleep efficiency, and overall mental health.

- **Other benefits of participating in a regular tai chi exercise program include:** reducing prenatal anxiety and depression, reducing chronic pain, reducing the symptoms of fibromyalgia, stroke, osteoarthritis, heart failure, and rheumatoid arthritis. Tai chi practice may also benefit cardiovascular fitness.

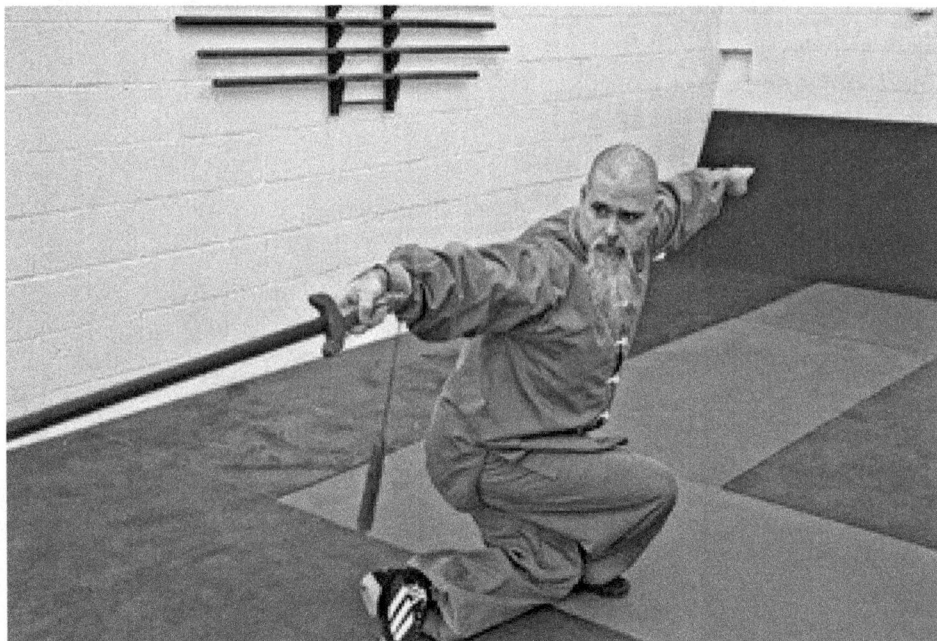

Tai Chi Sword

The Tai Chi Salutation

Classes and forms normally begin and end with courtesy expressed through what we refer to as the "salutation". It is essentially the martial arts version of a handshake. This is performed by placing your right fist into your left palm, facing the person or thing you are paying respect to, and bending slightly at the waist but keeping your eyes up.

This salutation can also be done as a sign of respect to your instructor, your peers, or other students, as well as in other situations. The closed fist covered with an open hand symbolizes that you are not holding a weapon and implies that you come in peace.

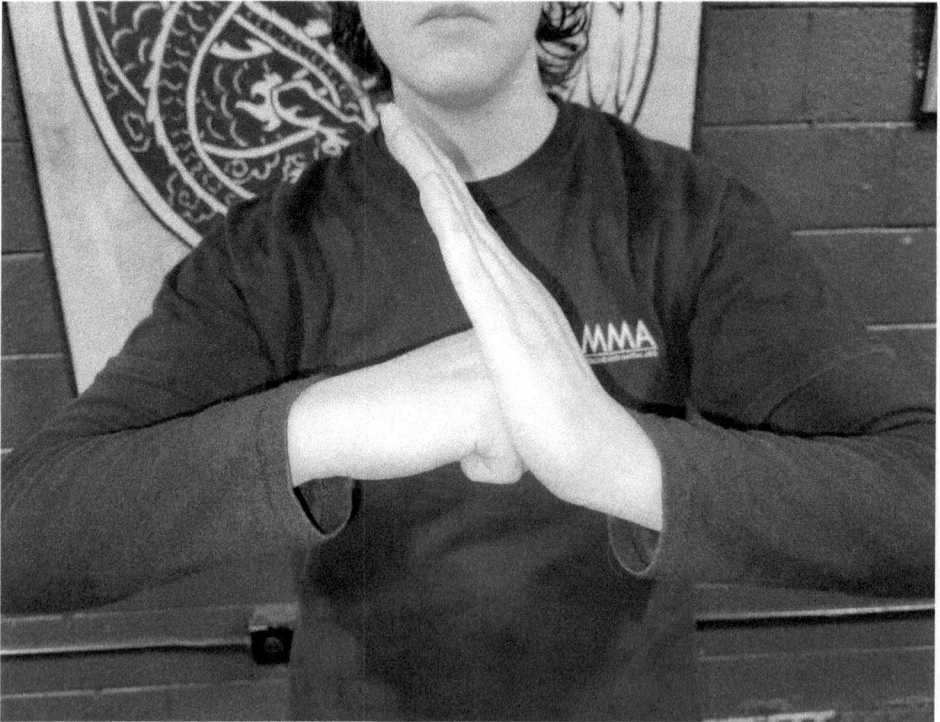

Tai Chi Salutation

Tai Chi Theory

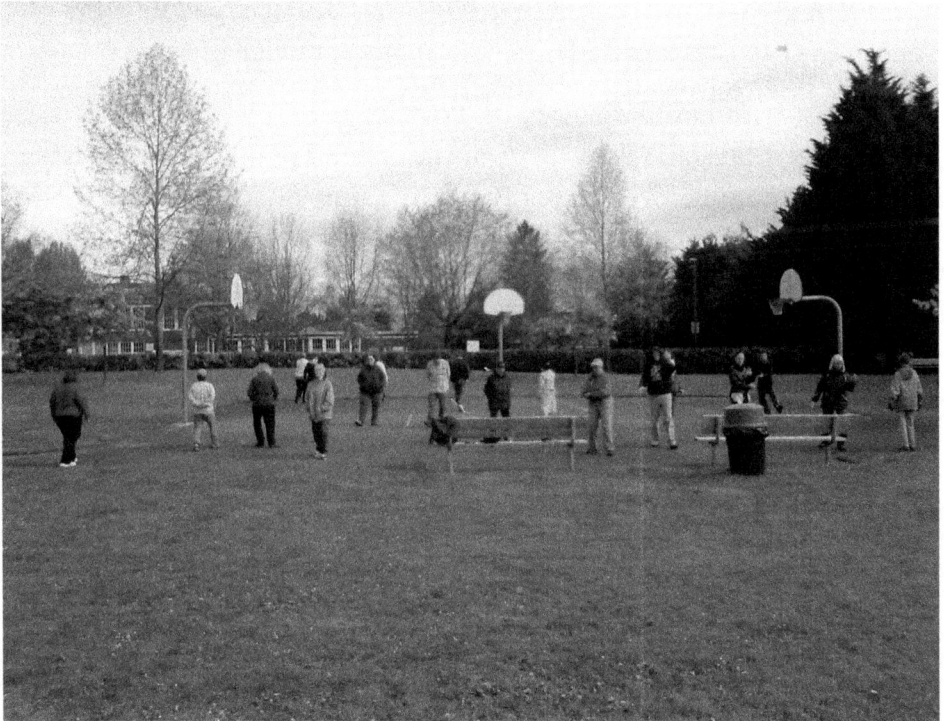

Tai Chi Practice

Virgil Flaim Park, Seattle

2014

The Cosmology of Tai Chi

Since the dawn of time, humans have looked into the night sky and wondered what does it all mean. In antiquity ancient Chinese scholars, mystical Taoist masters, and insightful shaman developed theories about the origins of the universe and our role in it. One enduring theory postulates that the cosmos is governed and regulated by the Tao. The Tao can refer to the nameless and structureless universe or it can refer to a method of living in accordance with it. A great deal of Chinese thought has been shaped or influenced by Taoism to include the theory and practice of tai chi.

Tai chi is based on the theory of *Yin/Yang* and follows an ancient cosmology that starts with *wu ji,* or the state of potential that existed the moment before the Big Bang. In Taoist philosophy, *wu ji* refers to our "original nature". In tai chi it is sometimes stated that from *wu ji* (unity), comes the "ten thousand things". We start our tai chi practice from the position of attention or stillness. This stillness mirrors the *wu ji.* With our first movement, we create *yin* and *yang* and set them into motion. This motion continues unabated until the end of the practice when we return to stillness, entering into the state of *wu ji,* where all actions once again become pure potential. Our tai chi practice is a microcosm of the vibrations of the universe. Tai chi is less about "tapping into" this vibration and more about developing an awareness that we are, in fact, never separate from it. We strive to feel this connectivity with every step and with every breath.

During practice, try to quiet your mind. Let the energies coursing through your body resonate with the energies of the universe. Our mantra is breathe and relax. Each breath brings *qi* into our body. We relax to facilitate the flow of *qi* and to better experience it. We differentiate movement and stillness, fastness and slowness, and rising and sinking, to better understand the difference between *yin* and *yang.*

We breathe in harmony with *yin* and *yang*, exhaling as we move forward and inhaling as we move back.

Through practice, we strive to improve our physical body and health, our vital energy, and eventually, our spirit.

Components of Tai Chi

There are many activities that could be included in the practice of tai chi. It has been around long enough that innumerable gifted instructors from around the world have contributed to its legacy. One school's curriculum may be different from another school's. Some may stress the importance of health, some may emphasize martial applications and weapons forms. Still others may prioritize spiritual development, community, or stress management. The following are the components emphasized in the author's school:

- **Relaxation and breath training**
- **Cultivation and circulation of** *qi*
- **Rooting**
- **Empty hand forms**
  - Simplified Form (24-move)
  - Traditional Form (108-move)
- **Push hands and sensitivity training**
- **Weapons forms** (sword, saber, spear, and fan)
- *Jing*/**power development**
- **Qi gong and health cultivation practices**
  - Tai Chi Qi Gong (18-move/Shibashi)
  - Qi Coiling Gong
  - Minor Universal Circulation Qi Gong
  - Dao Yin (longevity practices)
  - Tai Chi Walking
  - Acupressure
- *Dao yin*/**longevity practices**
- **Tai chi theory** (*qi*, *yin*/*yang*, five elements, etc.)

What is Qi?

How we define *qi* in large part depends on the type of lens we use to examine it. *Qi* is both form and function, matter and energy. It exists inside of us while simultaneously permeating the outside spaces. It forms a continuum from the most far-flung galaxies to the molecules in our bodies. It is vibration.

Qi comes from the air we breathe and the food we consume. It can also be cultivated through the practice of qi gong. Although the best practice is to refer to it as "*qi*", we may call it "life force" or "energy", and although inaccurate, it is close enough to meet our needs. When our *qi* is healthy, we are healthy. When our *qi* becomes stagnant or inadequate, we may become sick.

The Chinese character for *qi* depicts elements of steam emanating from a bowl of rice; with this one image, it is possible to intuit how *qi* is simultaneously substantive (the rice in the bowl) while at the same time insubstantial (the rising steam and the nourishment potential contained in the rice). From the perspective of Traditional Chinese Medicine (TCM), *Qi* is manufactured in the Spleen (an energetic function of TCM physiology) from the food and drink that we consume. If the quality of your air or food is poor or inadequate, your *qi* will suffer. *Qi* is stored in the lower abdomen and carried through energetic channels in your body. Tai chi attempts to circulate the *qi* through these channels for optimal health. *Qi* can also be accessed through specific points on your body via the insertion of fine needles into acupuncture points. We will sometimes massage these points to help regulate or stimulate the *qi* using acupressure techniques.

Breath is intimately connected to our *qi*, so both tai chi and qi gong have many methods and styles of breathing to accomplish different objectives.

Consequences to Qi Imbalances

For maximum health, Traditional Chinese Medicine (TCM) teaches us that harmoniously flowing *qi* of sufficient amount is required. When out of balance, *qi* tends to become stagnant, an excess condition characterized by erratic flow through the body, or deficient, characterized by too little *qi* for proper function. Stagnant *qi* conditions tend to result in pain, while deficient *qi* conditions tend to result in fatigue or hypo-functioning of one's internal organs. Both qi gong and tai chi can help one regain harmony and balance with their *qi*.

The Five Spirits

Our physical existence is guided and enriched by five internal and intangible aspects known as *wu shen*, which are experienced by us all, and yet remain difficult to describe. In our paradigm, these five are the Spirit of the Heart (*shen*), Spirit of the Kidney (*zhi*), Spirit of the Spleen (*yi*), Spirit of the Lung (*p'o*), and the Spirit of the Liver (*hun*). Briefly, *shen* manifests the psychological, spiritual, and emotional parts of our lives. *Zhi* is our willpower, which is intimately tied to addiction. *Yi* is our intention. *P'o* is our corporeal body, it is the part of us that returns to the earth when we die. *Hun* is our ethereal body; when our bodies eventually fade the *hun* lives on, exiting our bodies at the acupuncture point known as "Hundred Meetings", for the constellation "Big Dipper".

These five spirits are directly influenced by the quality of our *qi*, and in turn, when these Spirits become imbalanced they can affect our *qi* and our health. The practice of tai chi can help keep their energies from becoming stagnant and causing disease.

Shen and Yi and their Relevance to Tai Chi

Yi is a Chinese word that means, among other things, intention. It is one of the "*wu shen*" or "five spirits". In TCM, *yi* is governed by the Spleen. This means that disharmony to the Spleen will negatively impact your *yi*. *Yi* is related to thinking, processing, and problem-solving. We say that "*yi* leads *qi*". This means that if you want your *qi* to go somewhere you must lead it there with the *yi*. We sometimes use tapping or pressure to help *yi* bring *qi* to a specific area. When we want *qi* to circulate from one place to another it is our *yi* that allows it to happen. When *yi* is leading *qi* correctly, our tai chi postures and movements are alive and our strikes are more effective.

Closely related to *yi* is *shen*, the Spirit of the Heart. *Shen* is related to what the Western world might think of as "spirit". In tai chi, any time we use our "mind's eye" to look inside of ourselves, it is our *shen* that facilitates this. While practicing, our head and eyes should be moving just in front of our *yang* hand (the action hand) to properly direct the *yi* and *shen*.

What is Yin/Yang Theory?

This is a core theory of tai chi. Fundamentally, *yin/yang* theory is a way of describing how two things relate to each other. Understanding *yin* and *yang* are essential to understanding and improving your tai chi practice. It is a way to look at, interpret, and understand the universe, through a very definitive and limiting set of five rules or laws.

This theory suggests that there is a dynamic, ongoing relationship between two paired things. When you punch at me, my response creates this relationship. *Yin/yang* theory gives us the principles we use to defend. Instead of blocking your attack I move in harmony with it, deflecting your energy and letting it move you to a compromised position that I can then exploit.

The Five Laws of Yin/Yang

The five laws of *yin/yang* theory are **1.** opposition, **2.** mutual generation and support, **3.** infinite divisibility, **4.** interdependence, and **5.** inter-transformation. Although an in-depth discussion of this theory is beyond the scope of this book, your tai chi practice must conform to these laws. Tai chi is the physical and energetic manifestation of *Yin/Yang* Theory and a practical, functional understanding of this theory is a requirement for mastery.

- **Opposition.** A *yin/yang* pairing must be opposite each other for the comparison to make sense. For example hot/cold, light/dark, high/low. It is only through their opposing nature that yin/yang can be revealed. This opposition both restricts and controls.

- **Mutual Generation and Support.** A *yin/yang* pairing must contain the seed of its opposite. There must be a little bit of *yin* contained in a thing that is *yang*. We see this when prescribing Chinese herbs. If a patient is to be given a *Yang* Tonifying formula, it can not contain only *yang* tonic herbs; there must be some *yin* herbs in the formula as well to provide balance. They consume and create each other in a never-ending cycle.

- **Infinite Divisibility.** Any *yin/yang* phenomena must be able to be divided to make two smaller, but equal *yin/yang* phenomena. For example in a 24-hour day, we may describe 6am—6pm as the *yang* part of the day, and 6pm—6am as the *yin* part of the day. For this law to apply, I must be able to take either half of the above (let us use 6am—6pm), cut it in half, and make two new *yin/yang* pairings. So, 6am-12pm will become *yang*, and 12pm-6pm will become *yin*. And so on in either direction.

- **Interdependence**. *Yin* and *yang* phenomena have no meaning until compared and contrasted with each other. Nothing exists in a vacuum. To say that a building is tall is meaningless until there is a shorter building to compare it to. At that point "tall" becomes a contextualized, usable piece of information.

- **Inter-transformation**. *Yin* and *yang* phenomena must be able to transform into each other. Day turns to night, night turns to day. It is a dynamic and continuous process.

The chart below shows the *yin/yang* symbol with its representative components.

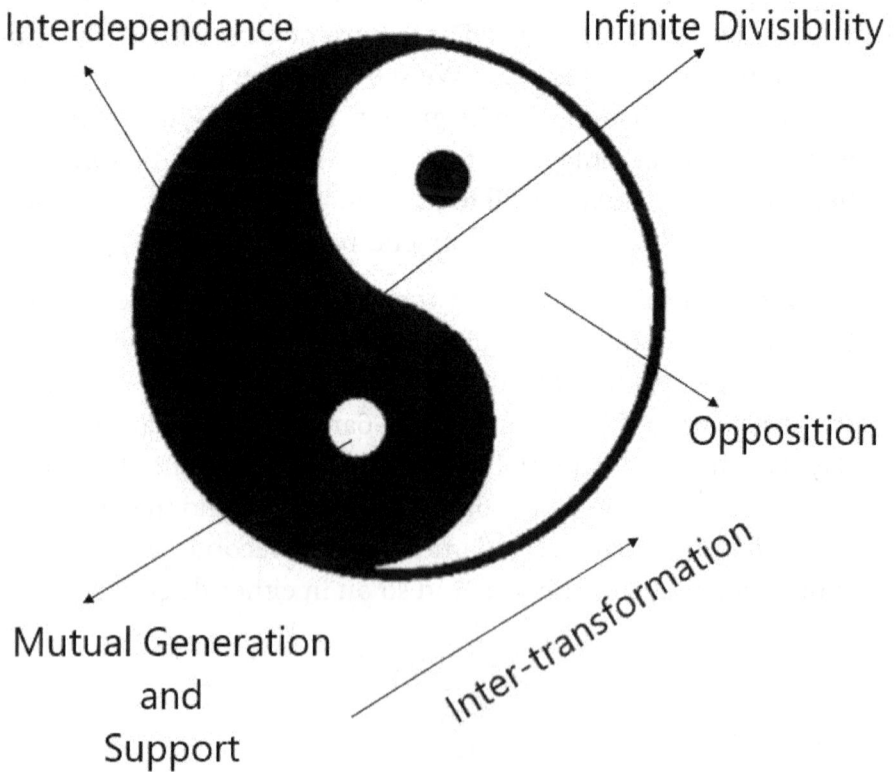

Interdependance

Infinite Divisibility

Opposition

Mutual Generation
and
Support

Inter-transformation

Five Laws of *Yin/Yang*

How do Yin and Yang Manifest in Tai Chi?

Yang movements are forward, upward, offensive in nature, or move in a straight line. *Yin* movements are backwards, downwards, defensive in nature, or circular. Movements that are fast are *yang* in nature, and movements that are slow are *yin* in nature. Additionally, movements that are hard or forceful are *yang,* and movements that are soft or yielding are *yin.*

Yin and *yang* show a relationship between two things. They are not absolutes. For instance, it's not correct to describe the speed of a car as fast, and therefore is yang. Rather, the speed of the car is yang relative to the speed of a slower moving bicycle.

We can use this theory for tai chi fighting applications and push hands. When our partner pushes straight at us hard in an attempt to disrupt our balance (*yang*), we can softly yield, turning his force out to dissipate his energy (*yin*).

What Does it Mean to Cultivate Qi?

Cultivating *qi* is the process of renewing the volume of available *qi* in your body. It includes breathing, visualization, active mind exercises, and working with the *tan tien*. Other factors can be involved such as physical movements or exercises, colors, sounds, or vibrations. Additionally, diet and nutrition, sleep, overall health, acupuncture, herbs, and other activities of daily living (ADL) can play an important part.

Qi Sensation

Qi sensation is the physical feeling of the energy in your body. These feelings can represent a healthy or unhealthy sensation. In health, the *qi* sensation may feel dull and achy, warm, moving, tingly, or heavy. These indicate the harmonious movement of *qi* and connection. Negative sensations manifest as cold, sharp, painful, or focused on a specific area. These feelings indicate that the *qi* is not flowing correctly, that it is stagnant or deficient.

Tan Tien

The *tan tien* is an insubstantial place located in your lower abdomen, between your kidneys and your abdominal muscles. The *tan tien* has two principal functions. The first is an energetic function - it acts like a battery to store your body's *qi*. The second is a physiological function – it is your body's center of gravity. This is particularly important in maintaining balance, facilitating correct movement, directing power, and self-defense.

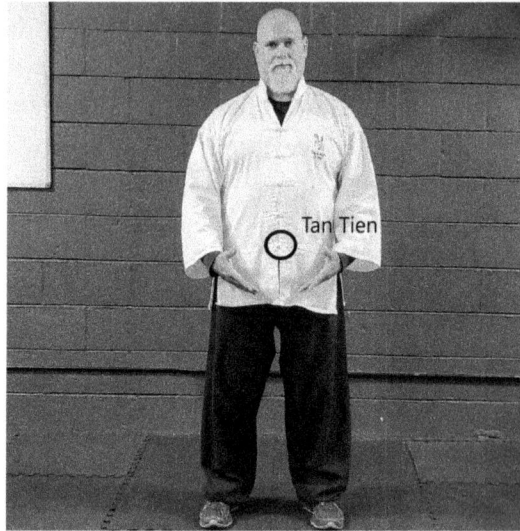

Tan Tien

Five Elements Theory

Five Elements Theory is a method of describing how phenomena relate to each other. Whereas *Yin/Yang* Theory is excellent at describing how two things interact and relate to each other at a macro or cosmic level, Five Elements Theory allows for more complex relationships to be described and is better at explaining how more tangible things relate at the temporal or micro level. Although often translated as "elements" it is sometimes helpful to think of it instead as "movements" or "phases". The elements are Fire, Earth, Metal, Water, and Wood. For our purposes in tai chi, the Five Elements can relate to movement, where Metal is a forward moving energy, Earth represents a central equilibrium, Wood is a retrograde or backwards moving energy, Water is movement (or awareness) to the left, and Fire is movement (or awareness) to the right. Additionally, the Five Elements are a way of thinking about responding to external stimuli or they can be thought of as stance, footwork, and fighting strategy. When applied to fighting strategy, Fire moves forward and up, Earth is energy that moves through the center, often circling or spiraling, Wood expands outward, Water sinks and moves backwards, and Metal brings things together.

The Five Elements as Movement

These are the classical movement directions or footwork in tai chi.

- Forward (Metal)

- Backward (Wood)

- Left (Water)

- Right (Fire)

- Center (Earth)

The Five Elements as Martial Theory

An alternative way to think about tai chi martial theory, the following can be either offensive or defensive. The Five Elements Form (described on pages 166-173) makes use of these maneuvers, bridging the gap between theory and practice.

- To bring two things together, to synthesize (Metal). This is seen in movements like Play the Peipa.

- To expand outward (Wood). This is seen in movements like Single Whip.

- To sink or move backwards (Water). This is seen in movements like Step Back and Repulse Monkey.

- To rise or move forward (Fire). This is seen in movements like Grasp Sparrow's Tail.

- Center (Earth). This is seen in movements like Step Up, Deflect, Parry, and Punch.

The Generating Cycle

The Generating Cycle is one way of showing the relationship between elements. In this theory, Fire generates Earth, Earth generates Metal, Metal generates Water, Water generates Wood, and
Wood generates Fire allowing the cycle to begin again. We can tell a
story as it pertains to the Five Elements moving through the Generating Cycle.

A campfire burns down, and its ashes mix with the ground, soon
becoming impossible to separate from the earth. When the earth is
dug into, metals can be extracted. These metals can be shaped into
tools. When these tools are left outside overnight, condensation can
form. The water from the condensation can be used to nurture
plants. Trees can be hewn into wood, which in turn can be used to
make fire, beginning the cycle anew. Other relationships between
the Five Elements exist but are not as relevant to the practice of tai
chi.

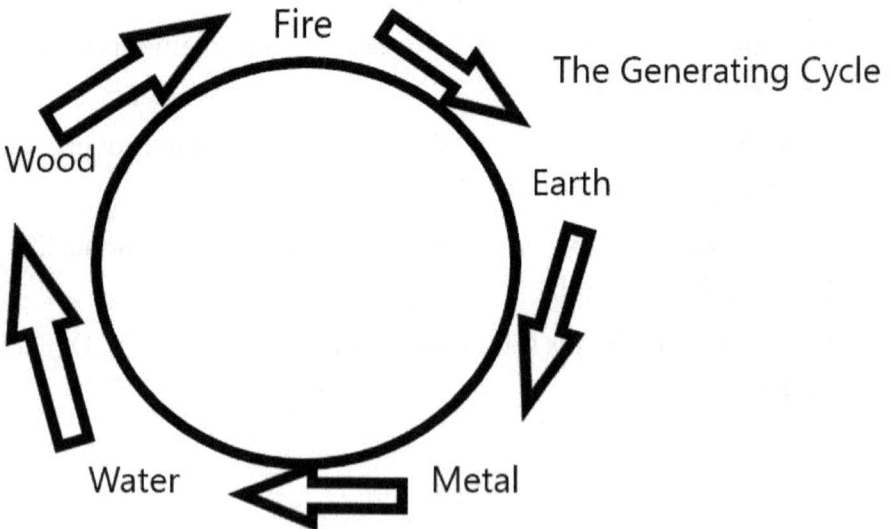

Fire

Wood

The Generating Cycle

Earth

Water

Metal

Acupressure Points

There are a few specific acupressure points on the body that it will be helpful to be able to find. These points can be useful for health maintenance, to emit *qi*, or to strike an opponent during combat. The following points are among the most important for our practice (point location is indicated with a green dot):

- **Pericardium (PC) 8.** Located in the palm between the 2nd and 3rd metacarpal bones. When a loose fist is made the point will be found where the tip of the middle finger rests. Used to emit *qi* when striking with the palm. It is also used to clear heat from the Heart.

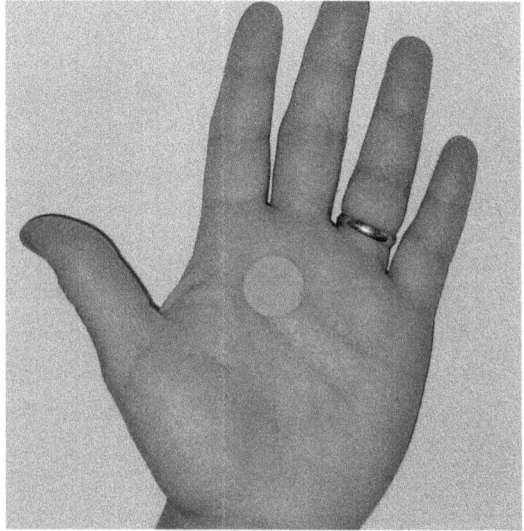

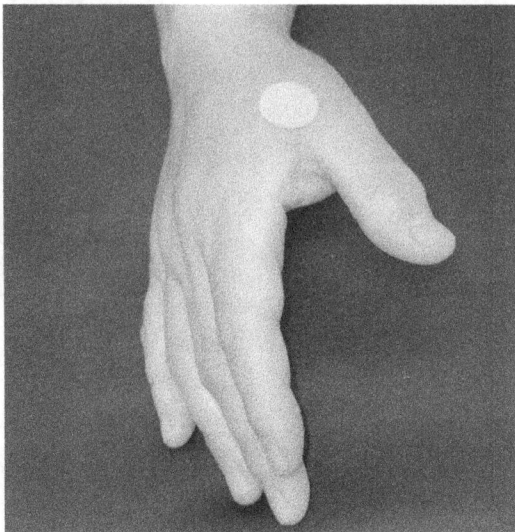

- **Large Intestine (LI) 4.** Located on the hand in the fleshy area between the thumb and the index finger. This is one of the most useful acupuncture points. Used for stopping a variety of painful conditions of the head and face (like toothaches or earaches). It is an excellent point to massage for headaches. It is also good for moving stagnant *qi*.

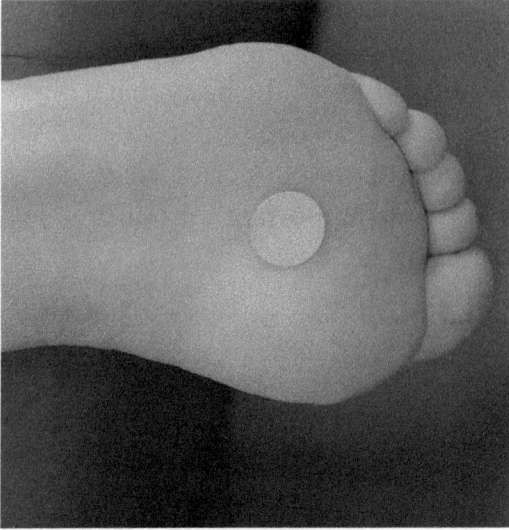

- **Kidney (KD) 1.** Located on the bottom of the foot at approximately the top one third of the foot. Sink your *qi* into the ground through this point to root. It can be massaged when someone has fallen unconscious to help revive them. It can also be massaged to help calm someone down and treat anxiety. To get a tangible sense of this points value in movement and balance, contrast shifting your weight between the balls of your feet and your heels. You will immediately feel the difference. When the weight is over your heels you will feel awkward and unbalanced. With your weight over this point you will feel stable and in a balanced position to respond to an outside stimulus.

- **Stomach (ST) 36.** Located on the side of the leg below the knee and one fingers width lateral to the tibia bone. One of the most important points to tonify *qi* and promote general wellness. It also can reduce fatigue and have a positive effect on digestion. Known as "Leg Three Miles" because Chinese soldiers in antiquity knew to massage it while on bivouac to get the energy to walk three more miles.

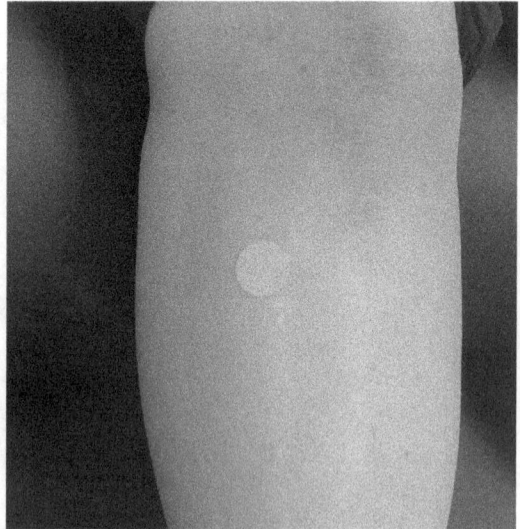

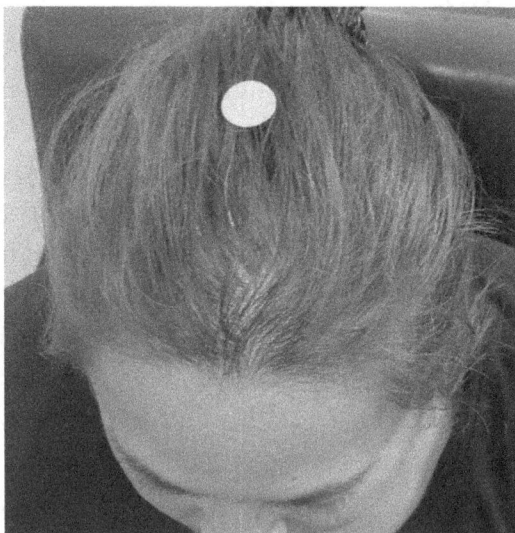

- **Governing (DU) 20**. Located at the top of the head, this point is used to expel bad *qi* when doing qi gong. It can be massaged to help alleviate symptoms of vertigo or dizziness, and can be helpful to clear the mind.

Three Taoist Treasures

In Traditional Chinese Medicine, the Three Taoist Treasures are *Jing*, *Qi*, and *Shen*. These are the essential components of life. Loosely translated it can be thought of as mind, body, and spirit, where *jing* is your physical body, *qi* is your vital force, and *shen* is the various manifestation of your psychology, spirituality, and emotions. How does tai chi facilitate this development? Through mindful and consistent practice.

In the beginning, tai chi practice focuses on exercises and drills that strengthen the body and improve overall feelings of health and wellbeing. This is the first Treasure.

Over time, students are taught how to integrate breathing into their movements, establish a solid root, circulate internal energy, and bring qi to their *tan tien*. This is the second Treasure.

The third Treasure is to use your tai chi practice to cultivate a more mindful and spiritual path.

Jing

Jing can be thought of as power generation based on a combination of physics, mechanics, and internal energy. It is also an understanding of how to efficiently use your body to transfer power from the ground to your target. It can be contrasted with "*li*", or muscle power, a type of power that we do not want in tai chi. Although *jing* uses muscles, it is more than just muscle power. *Jing* originates in the ground (shaped and guided into your body through your feet), transfers to your *tan tien* via your tendons and ligaments, and is supported by *qi*. With no root, there is no *jing*. As you age, *li* fades but *jing* can stay strong and vital.

Jing can manifest in different ways—it can be offensive, defensive, explosive, hard, or soft. With proper body alignment and mental focus, *jing* becomes alive and fluid, whereas *li* stays stagnant. *Jing* is rounded, smooth, and reactive to your intention, *li* is square, jagged, and unresponsive. Yet another way to conceptualize the difference between these two types of power is that *li* floats to the surface while *jing* sinks into the ground through your root.

If there is a secret to the power of tai chi, it is in the study of *jing*. Truly, our pursuit of skill in the study of tai chi is in developing an understanding of how relaxation and proper body alignment opens up the opportunity to express *jing*.

A variety of drills are used to practice and develop *jing*. The best way to understand *jing* is through a partner drill known as push hands.

Developing *jing* takes time and it incorporates many skills; relaxation, proper breathing, root, sensitivity, power expression, kinetic linking, and many more. Training advances through four stages, starting with listening. Listening is the skill of staying in contact with your partner while performing technique. Over time listening turns to understanding.

Understanding is being able to interpret what you are listening to and formulate a coherent and directed reaction. Neutralizing is manifesting the response to affect your partner's attack, and emitting is implementing your response or counterattack.

Broadly speaking there are four categories of *jing* development:

- **Listening.** Consists of sticking or adhering to your partner as they move and attack. It is only by staying in contact that it will be possible to feel their tension. It is a prerequisite for all of the other *jing* skills. This skill can be trained with a hanging target or with a partner, and it consists of learning how to maintain physical contact and staying soft and relaxed while doing so.

- **Understanding.** Through practice and repetition, it is possible to read the intention of your partner and interpret their potential actions. When they change direction, increase or decrease the force in their attack, or maneuver, you will eventually be able to feel it and use this information to make your own response.

- **Neutralizing.** This is the process of countering your partner's movements. When they attack, we yield. When they retreat, we can follow or disrupt their movements.

- **Emitting.** This is the projection of energy back into your partner; your counterattack.

Wu Ji

This is an ancient Taoist philosophical concept that appears as far back as the 4th century BCE. It shows up in a book called the **Tao Te Ching** and has many shades of meaning. It can refer to infinity, a state of unity, or nothingness. It is the moment before the Big Bang where everything exists in a state of pure potential.

In the form when you are standing still before you start, you are, if only symbolically, in a state of *wu ji*. We take a moment to clear our minds, feel the ground beneath our feet, and bring awareness to our *tan tien*. From *wu ji*, you begin the form and create a separation of *yin* and *yang* through movement and intention. At the end of the form, you return to a state of *wu ji*.

Breathing

The ancients noted that babies breathe low in their bellies and the elderly breathe high in their chests. Subsequently, they associated long life and health with breathing low into the *tan tien*, working the abdomen like a bellows.

Breathing is an art and a science, and there are many systems, methods, and styles of breathing. The cultivation of internal energy (*qi*) is intimately connected to breathing, as is the generation of power. Without breath, there is neither *qi* nor life. Breathing is so fundamental to the practice of tai chi, that it is accurate to say that the only two *really* important skills to develop are breathing and relaxation.

There are two methods that a tai chi student should be aware of. The first is natural abdominal breathing. This is the style of breathing to be used by new tai chi students. It is very easy, simply place the tip of your tongue on the roof of your mouth and breathe naturally. Over time, begin to expand your abdomen with each inhalation, and contract your abdomen when you breathe out. Practice breathing low.

Once the student is more acclimated to their tai chi practice, it is appropriate to explore the second type of breathing; a more complicated breathing that conforms to the principles of *Yin/Yang* Theory. Generally, you can think of inhaling as storing *qi* and exhaling as emitting *qi*. When you move forward or down, exhale.

When you move backwards or up, inhale. When you separate your hands inhale. When you bring your hands together or move to strike, exhale. Never hold your breath while hitting something.

As a general rule, if you can hear your own breathing you are breathing too hard. Try to relax and slow your movements down to regulate your breath.

- *Tan Tien* **Breathing Exercise**. Adopt a small or traditional horse stance It is also acceptable to sit in a chair or on the floor, or to lie down. Place your hands either in front of or pressing into your *tan tien*. This will help your *yi* lead *qi* into your *tan tien*. Place your tongue on the roof of your mouth - this is done to connect the *Ren* and *Du* acupuncture channels to facilitate the flow of *qi*. Close your eyes and clear your mind. Focus on your breath. Inhale and expand your abdomen and bring *qi* into your body. With each exhalation, contract the muscles of your abdomen. As you exhale, guide *qi* into your *tan tien*. Connect your breath, body, and *qi* in your *tan tien*.

Relaxation

Learning to relax is one of the two most essential skills to develop in tai chi (the other is breathing). If you are tense it inhibits you from connecting your physical body to your energetic body. In addition to facilitating the smooth flow of *qi* in your body, other benefits of relaxation include: slowing your heart rate, lowering blood pressure, slowing your breathing rate, reducing the activity of stress hormones, increasing blood flow to major muscle groups, reducing muscle tension, alleviating chronic pain, improving concentration and mood, lowering fatigue, reducing anger and frustration, and boosting confidence.

Moreover, building time to relax into your daily schedule can help reduce long-term stress-related health issues.

Relaxation

The following describe a few specific relaxation techniques.

- **Internal thought focusing.** Think of a word or phrase that is positive and uplifting for you, then focus on it, repeating it to yourself. Be aware of your body and tell it to relax while performing this technique. This technique can be enhanced by turning your lips up in a slight smile. The act of smiling signals your body to release "feel good" chemicals like dopamine and serotonin.

- **Visualization.** Use your minds' eye to imagine that you are in a peaceful and happy place such as a forest or by the ocean. Imagine the sounds, smells, and physical sensations that go along with it. Like nearly every aspect of tai chi, this is a skill that will need to be acquired through practice. You may not be successful at visualization in the beginning but will get better over time.

- **Music.** Some students find that background music can help focus and quiet their minds to help them relax. A great deal of research exists detailing the various effects of different music on the mind.

- **Muscle tensing exercise.** This is a very effective technique for getting your muscles to relax, and for helping you to identify areas that are holding tension you might not have been aware of. The muscles need to be relaxed so that your *qi* can flow unimpeded. These can be done piecemeal or all of them can be done in a series. Tense the indicated muscle(s) and hold for 10 seconds then relax. Repeat as necessary. This exercise may show you what a relaxed muscle feels like so you know what sensation you are pursuing.

The following are examples of major muscle groups to relax with the above-described muscle tensing exercise:

- **Abdomen.** Flex the abdominal muscles and release.

- **Bicep curls.** Flex your bicep muscles as if you were curling a heavy weight, then release.

36

- **Buttocks.** Flex your glute muscles then release.

- **Chest.** Flex your pectoral muscles and release.

- **Eyes.** Squeeze your eyes shut then open.

- **Forearms.** Flex and relax the extensor and flexor muscles in the forearms.

- **Hands.** Clamp fists tightly and release

- **Jaw.** Clench your teeth together to flex the masseter muscle in your jaw, then release.

- **Plantar and dorsal flexion of feet.** Press your foot down as if stepping on the acceleration pedal in a car, then reverse.

- **Shoulders to ears.** Squeeze and press your shoulders up to your ears and hold. Release and exhale.

- **Toe curls.** Squeeze the muscles in your toes, do one foot at a time.

- **Thighs.** Flex and relax the large muscles in your thighs.

Song (or sung)

This is a tai chi term for deep relaxation or flow. It is the goal of our relaxation and forms training. This concept is found in many martial arts and is suggestive of the acquisition of what is commonly thought of as an "internal" skill (as opposed to an 'external' skill such as a punch or kick). One way that a person who has acquired "*song*" is described is as "steel wrapped in cotton". When you push on them they initially feel soft but as you sink into them you find that they are quite strong and rooted. *Song* also implies a method of responding to an external stimulus that does not result in conflict. For instance, we don't really "block" in tai chi, rather, we redirect, deflect, and parry an incoming strike or push. It is also a form of respect; if someone wants to go through us, perhaps by trying to push or punch us, we politely step out of the way and let them. Our goal is to never give our opponent a target that can be hit. As soon as their attack touches us we gently guide their energy to a safer place.

The Thirteen Postures

The thirteen postures are the core theoretical underpinnings of tai chi. Without these postures, there can be no tai chi. From these postures are derived the movements, techniques, theory, and applications of tai chi. Note that these "postures" are not exactly set physical movements but rather a collection of principles or skills, that can be applied in many ways.

The postures are divided up into eight energies (sometimes referred to as "gates" or "treasures") inspired by the Eight Trigrams, and five movements derived from the Five Elements. The Eight Trigrams describe the eight natural phenomena of Taoist cosmology first identified in a book called the Classic of Changes, or **I Ching**. These are heaven, lake, fire, wind, water, mountain, earth, and thunder. These eight are also sometimes referred to as the "*bagua*".

Five Elements Theory dates back to antiquity and is fully developed by the end of the Han Dynasty (206 BCE-220 CE) in China. This theory has been applied to many different areas of study from astrology to martial arts and medicine. These elements are represented by Fire, Water, Earth, Wood, and Metal, and can be thought of as a way of describing how phenomena relate to each other. In tai chi, we also think about them as maneuvers or direction of movement.

The Eight Energies

- Elbow stroke
- Pluck
- Press
- Push

- Rollback
- Shoulder stroke
- Split
- Wardoff

The Eight Energies Explained

The following are often done in conjunction with movement and in combination with other martial techniques.

- **Elbow stroke** (*zou*). Short, straight, sideways, absorbing. A strike or deflection with your elbow, often done as your opponent presses into you with an attack. Seen in push hands practice and self-defense applications.

- **Pluck** (*cai*). Short, straight, downward, sideways. A grab and either a push or a pull. Step Back and Repulse Monkey.

- **Press** (*ji*). Long or short, round, forward. Press brings two energies together with a squeezing motion. Play the Peipa.

- **Push** (*an*). Long or short, round, upward, downward. Push is done to immobilize your opponent's energy, push or hold them down, or to bounce them away. Grasp Sparrow's Tail.

- **Rollback** (*lu*). Long or short, round, sideways, yielding. Rollback is done to turn an incoming energy and lead it past you. It has a "small" version and a "large" version. Grasp Sparrow's Tail.

- **Shoulder stroke** (*kau*). Short, straight, absorbing. Shoulder stroke is the application of your shoulder. Seen in push hands practice and self defense applications.

- **Split** (*lie*). Long or short, straight, breaking, opening, opposing. Split is used to turn an incoming force in a different direction. White Stork Spreads Wings.

- **Wardoff** (*peng*). Long, round, upward, expanding. Wardoff is often used to "bounce" an opponent away with your forearm. Often wardoff is preceded by the holding a ball posture. Grasp Sparrow's Tail.

The following represents my own understanding and experience. Some of my interpretations may be unorthodox. The Eight Energies can be quantified by:

- **Length.** Long or short. This gives you an idea as to how big the motion you are creating is. It may also refer to how committed the motion is. Yet another way to think about length is where and how deeply you want your power transfer to penetrate. If I strike my opponent with long power, bouncing him away, I may be out of position if I want to throw him. In this example, a short technique might be a better choice.

- **Shape.** Straight or rounded. This could refer to either how the energy is delivered or its effect.

- **Direction.** Upward, downward, forward, backward, outward, turning/deflecting, spiraling, or a combination of two directions such as forward and upward. Refers to both the direction your energy is emitted to and the direction you intend your opponent to move to.

- **Special qualities.** *Absorbing*—to take the force of an opponent's attack and guide it into the ground through your root. *Yielding*—to move backwards in response to an opponent's attack and dissipate the energy. *Breaking*—to disrupt the energy of your opponent's attack. *Opening*—to open up your opponent and make them vulnerable to a counterattack. *Expanding*—energy that moves from your center outward, which can be done to disrupt your opponent's energy or balance.

Tai Chi Warm Ups, Stretches, and Exercises

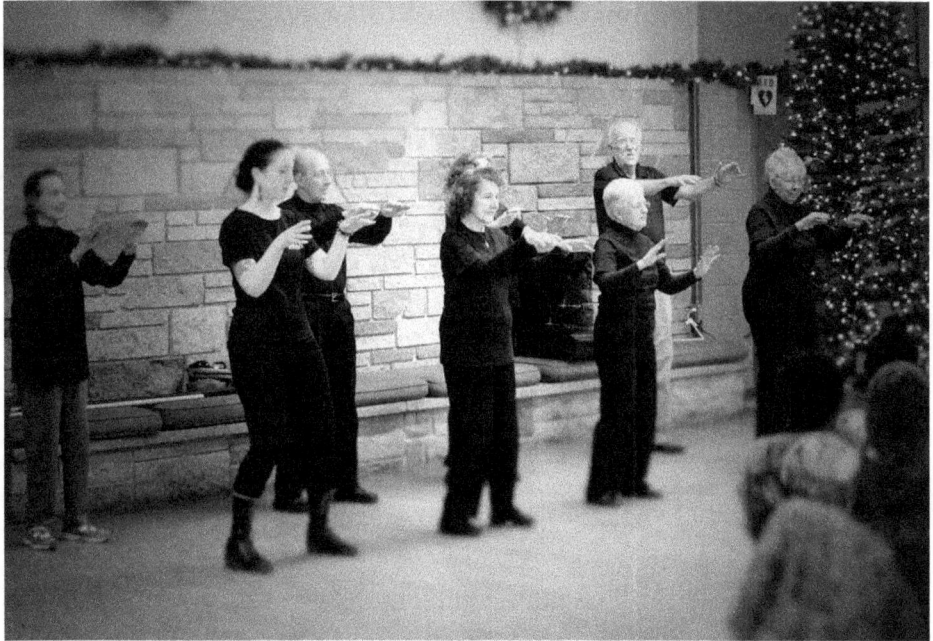

Tai Chi Performance

SAMMA End of Year Banquet

2017

Tai Chi Exercises

The stretches and warm-up exercises in tai chi are intended to prepare and condition your body for the specific requirements of the practice. They have a variety of functions that include maintaining or improving the student's overall health and fitness levels, cultivating and moving *qi*, and enhancing the student's understanding of specific tai chi techniques, movements, or principles. According to the Centers for Disease Control and Prevention (8), regular exercise can "...can improve your brain health, help manage weight, reduce the risk of disease, strengthen bones and muscles, and improve your ability to do everyday activities." Students often report being able to maintain or improve their flexibility level, enhanced feelings of wellbeing, improved mindfulness, reduced stress levels, and great benefit to their joints.

From the viewpoint of Traditional Chinese Medicine, tai chi can Regulate and Move Blood, Lubricate Joints, Calm *Shen*, Regulate Organ Function, Balance *Yin* and *Yang*, and Move *Qi* in the Meridians.

TCM Functions of Tai Chi Exercises Explained

- **Regulate and Move Blood.** When Blood doesn't move it results in a condition known as "Blood Stagnation" notable for inducing sensations of pain. The gentle and rhythmic motions found in tai chi exercises can activate blood and improve circulation.

- **Lubricate the Joints.** Tai chi exercises frequently focus on keeping *Qi* and Blood moving into and through the joints. When joints are appropriately lubricated they easily move through their natural range of motion without pain or inhibited mobility. Crepitus, or the cracking and crunching sounds some students hear while performing some exercises may be reduced through the practice of tai chi.

- **Calm *Shen***. *Shen* refers to your psychological, mental, and emotional state. Anxiety, worry, and stress can negatively impact your *shen*. Conscientiously performing the below exercises may bring an enhanced sense of wellbeing and stress reduction to the student. Exercise in general can have a positive impact on mental and emotional health.

- **Regulate Organ Function**. Many of these exercises' movements are targeted towards specific TCM organs. In particular the Spleen and Liver benefit immensely from tai chi exercises, improving digestion and reducing feeling of stress.

- **Move *Qi* in the Meridians**. Being sedentary increases the likelihood of experiencing *Qi* Stagnation. Exercise can assist the Liver in Moving the *Qi* and keeping Stagnation at bay. Stagnation is thought to be one of the primary causes of disease in Traditional Chinese Medicine.

- **Balance *Yin* and *Yang***. *Yin* and *yang* are essential energies in our bodies and they are subject to conditions of both excess and deficiency. The movements of tai chi can balance *yin* and *yang*. For example, moves that are slow are thought to nourish *yin* and practicing tai chi in the morning can give your *yang* energy a boost.

Rotations

We begin each class with a series of rotational exercises. Rotations are applied to the neck, wrist, arm and shoulder, hip, knees, and ankles. Rotations are different than stretches. Stretches are targeted at improving the performance of muscles and tendons. Rotations are primarily performed to lubricate the joints. Joints are poorly vascularized, meaning that they are somewhat limited in blood supply. To combat this. many natural body movements force the joints to act as a pump to bring blood in, and this helps to explain why a sedentary lifestyle may be the root cause of some disease. An active lifestyle supported by rotational exercises can help keep joints mobile and may help maintain health and reduce morbidity.

In TCM we believe that everywhere you have an articulating joint is a natural place for your *qi* to get caught up and become stagnant. Stagnant *qi* causes disease. The gentle motions will open the channels and allow the *qi* to flow more harmoniously. They should not hurt while performing them. These should be performed slowly and without tension. Do 8-10 repetitions of each.

- **Arm and shoulder rotations. 1-4.** Circumduct the arm at the shoulder in each direction.

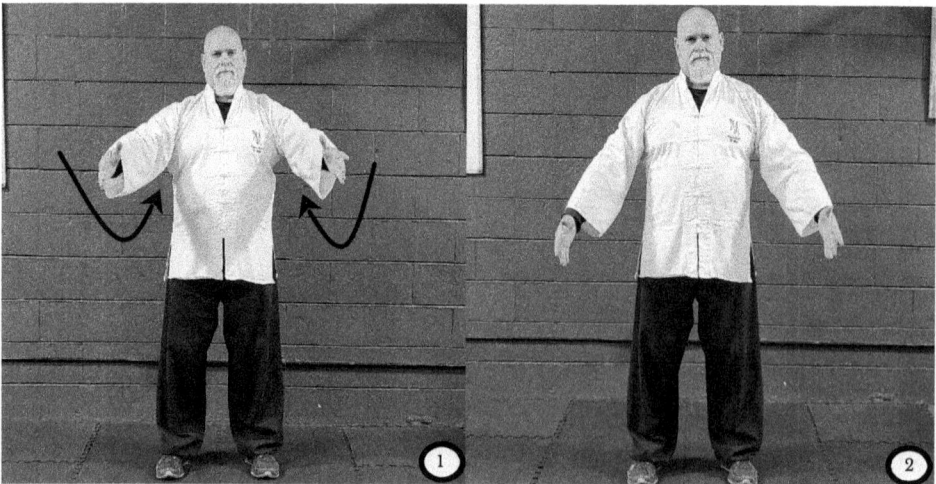

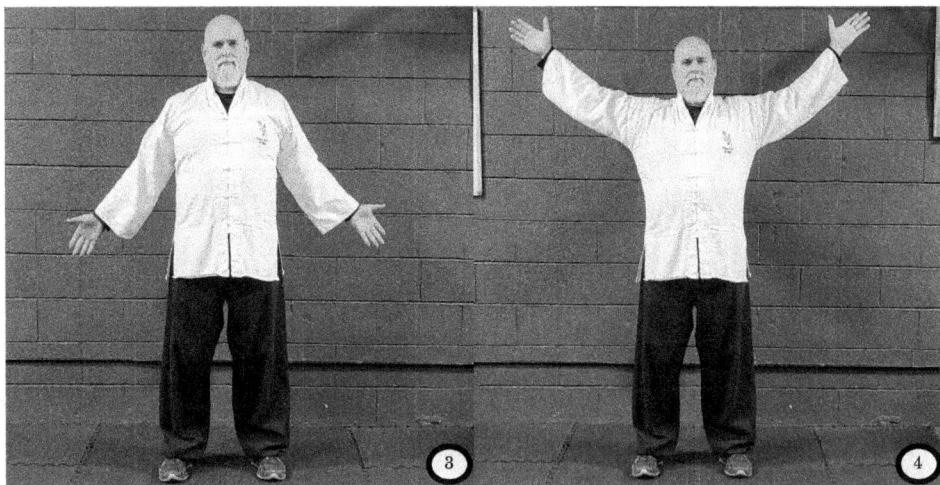

- **Elbow circles.** Hands held to front at chest level, palms up, pull arms back with your palms turned down, circle arms to the front, palms turn up.

- **Hip rotations.** **1.** Move your feet shoulder width apart. **2-5.** Put your hands on your hips and rotate the hip joint in each direction: forward, back, and side.

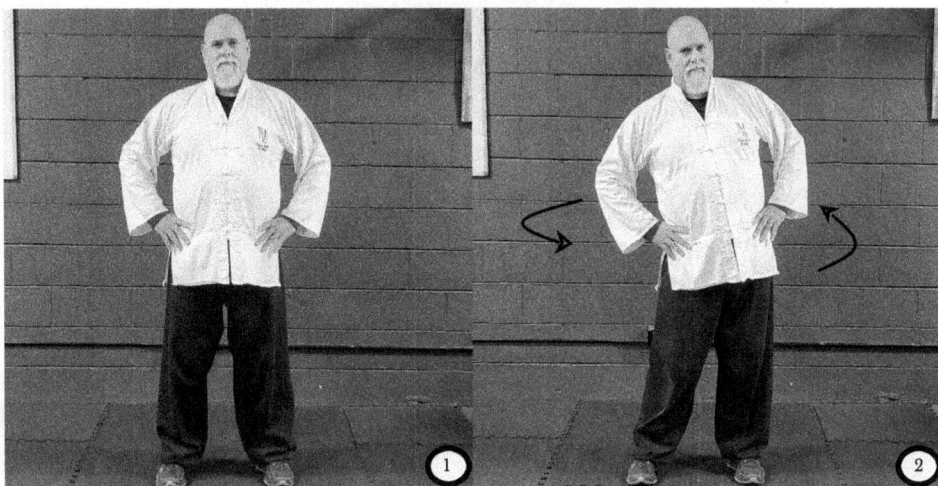

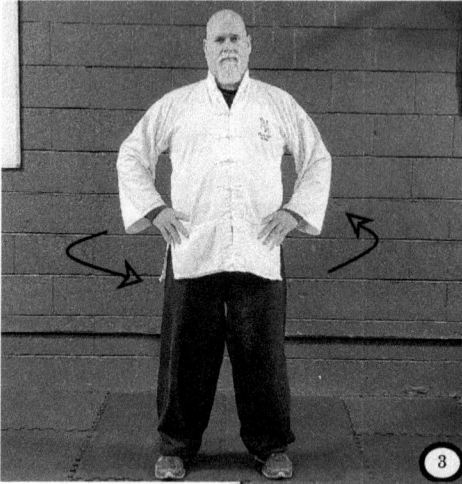

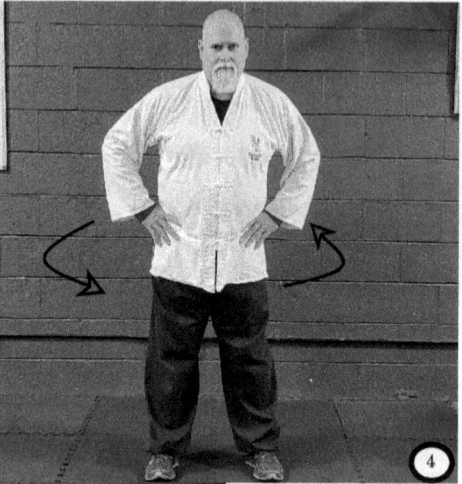

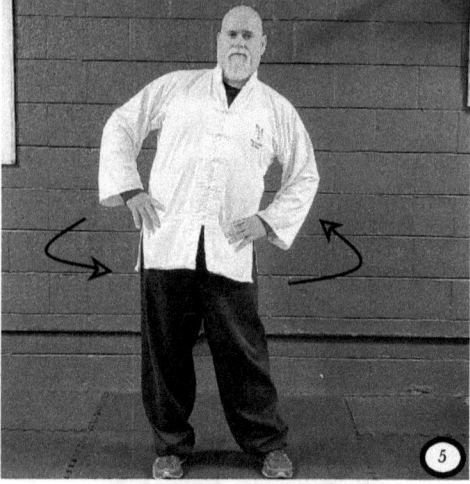

- **Knee and ankle rotations.** **1.** Bring your feet together and place your hands on your thighs, palms facing down, above the knee joints. (Note: Don't push down on the patella as this can cause injury when combined with knee rotation). **2-4.** Keep your knees slightly bent and rotate the knee and ankle joints through their range of motion.

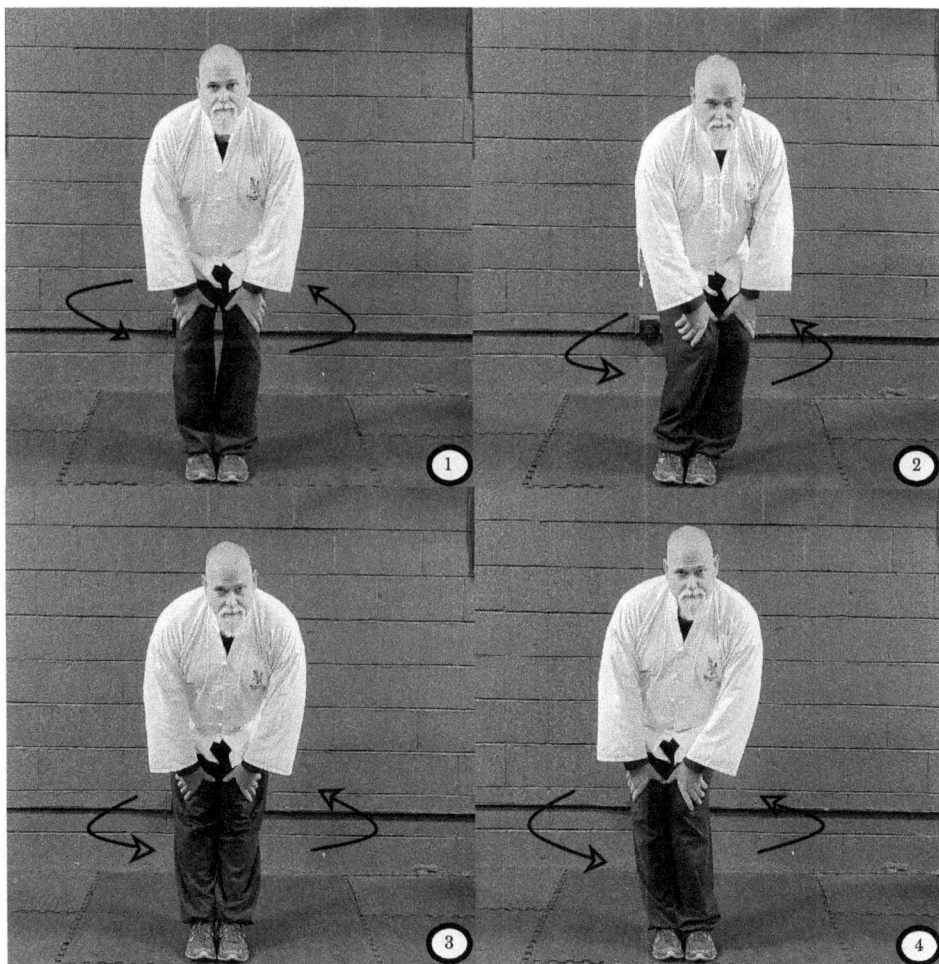

- **Neck rotations.** Rotate the neck joint in a circle. There is no need to make a large amplitude circle.

- **Nod head yes/shake head no.** Alternate flexing and extending the neck.

- **Wrist rotations.** Close your hands into fists and rotate wrists in both directions.

Stretches

A series of gentle stretches are normally done after performing rotations at the start of class. Stretches are done to prepare the soft tissue (muscles, tendons, ligaments, etc.) for safe tai chi practice. Stretching warms up and loosens the fascia, brings *qi* to the local area, and enhances blood flow to the muscles and tendons allowing them to work more efficiently. The act of stretching is to slowly extend the muscle towards its maximum length while avoiding any extreme motions. Do not bounce and do not move to the limits of a muscles range of motion too quickly. None of these stretches should hurt. A good rule of thumb is that if it hurts don't do it. Don't hold your breath or lock your knees while stretching. Hold each stretch for 10 to 60 seconds. Stretching can also be done at the end of class.

- **Abdominal stretch.** Legs are shoulder width apart. Interlock your fingers, extend your arms, and push your palms towards the ceiling. Once the arms are extended slightly move your hands backwards engaging your core.

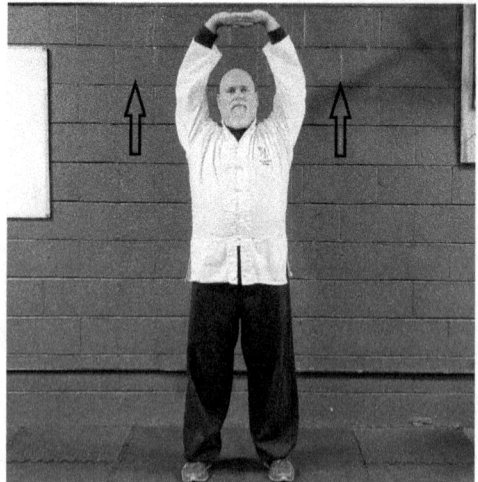

- **Circle the wrists. 1.** Clasp the hands together in front of your chest and interlock the fingers. **2-4.** Press the palms together and rotate the hands in a circle. Stretch through both directions.

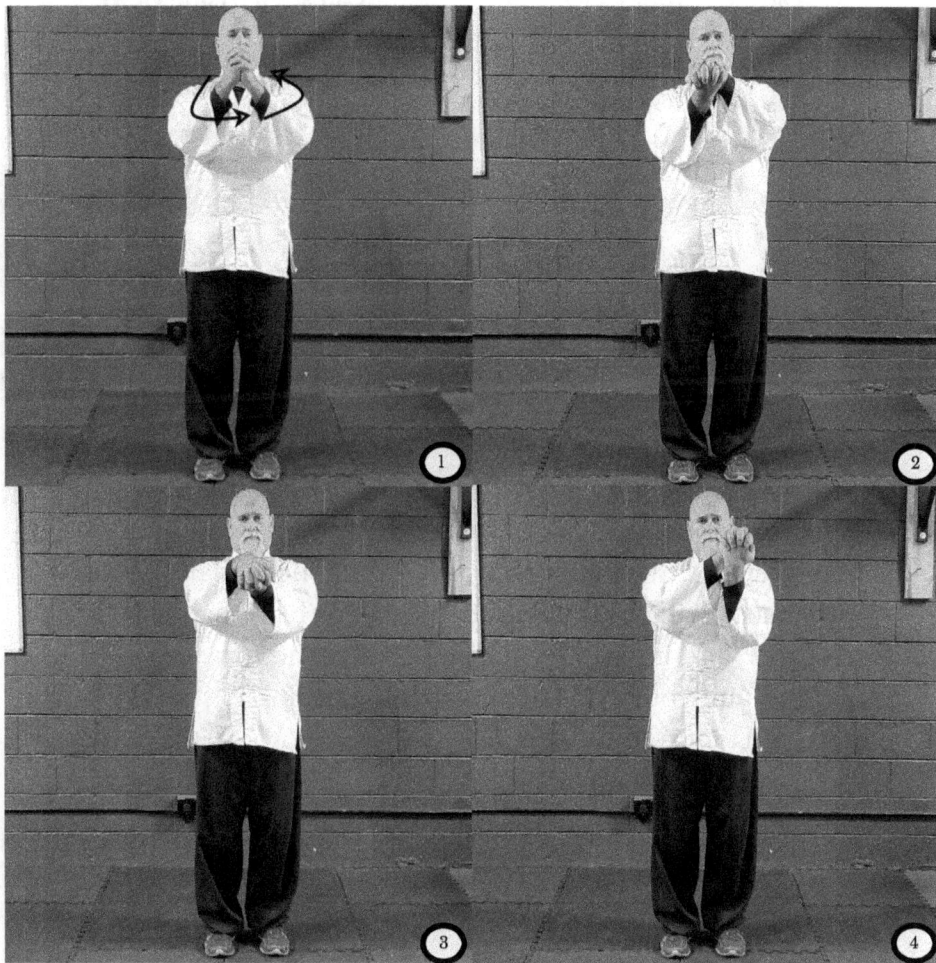

- **Calf stretch**. Step forward into a 60/40 stance. Push your back heel into the ground and bend your back knee until you feel the stretch in your back calf. Both of your feet should face forward.

Calf stretch (front view)   Calf stretch (side view)

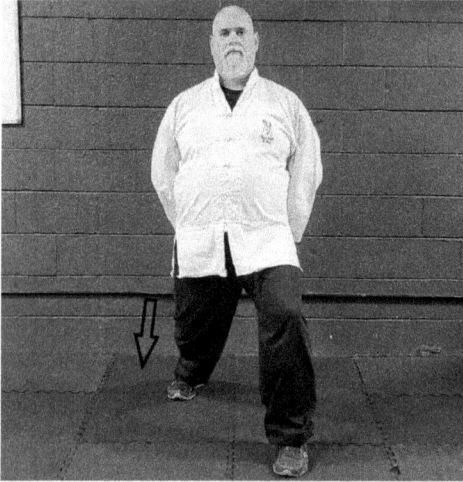

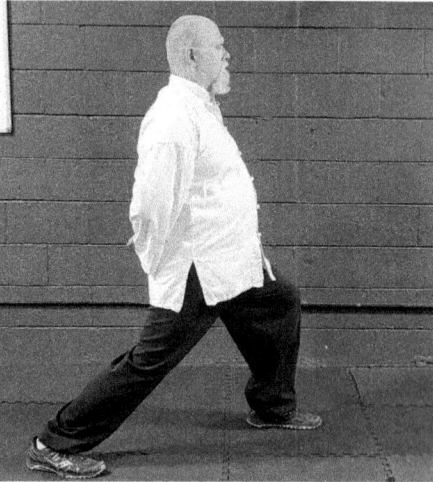

- **Chest stretch. 1.** Start with your feet a little more than shoulder width apart. Bring both hands behind your back, palms facing each other, and interlock your fingers. **2.** Bend forward at the waist and pull your arms up towards the ceiling to stretch your chest. Don't lock your knees.

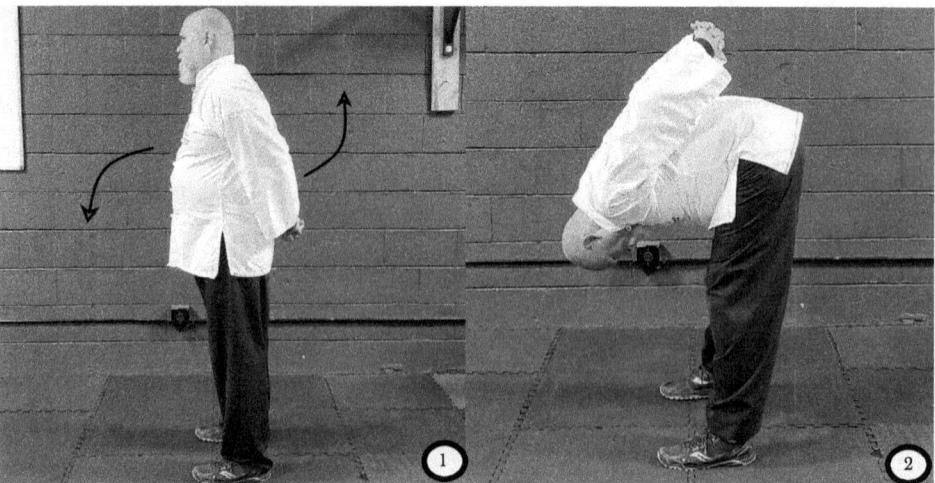

- **Elbow/shoulder circles**. **1**. Hands are held to the front of the abdomen. **2-3**. Back of hands touching, palms face out. Pull arms up, back of the hands are touching. **4-6**. Hands separate then move forward and down, circle arms to the back, bring hands forward until the back of the hands touch again. **7-8**. Bring hands back into the midline (held together), back of hands touching. Repeat.

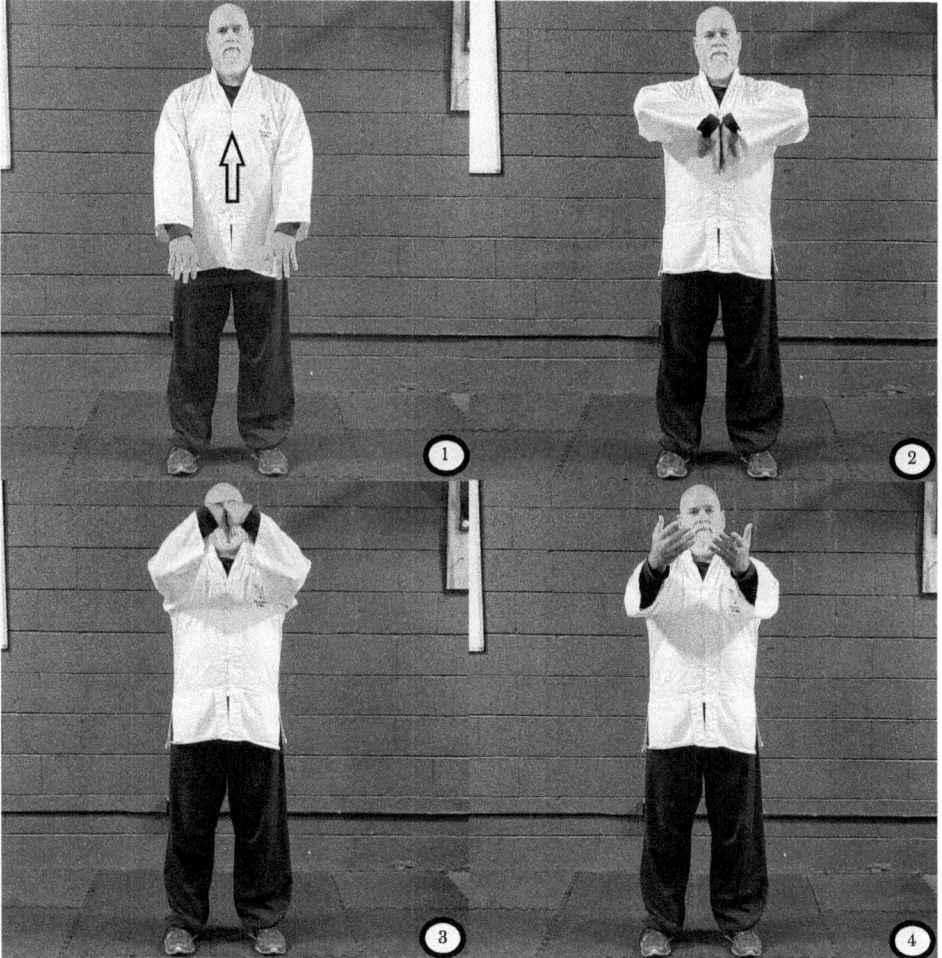

- Elbow/shoulder circles

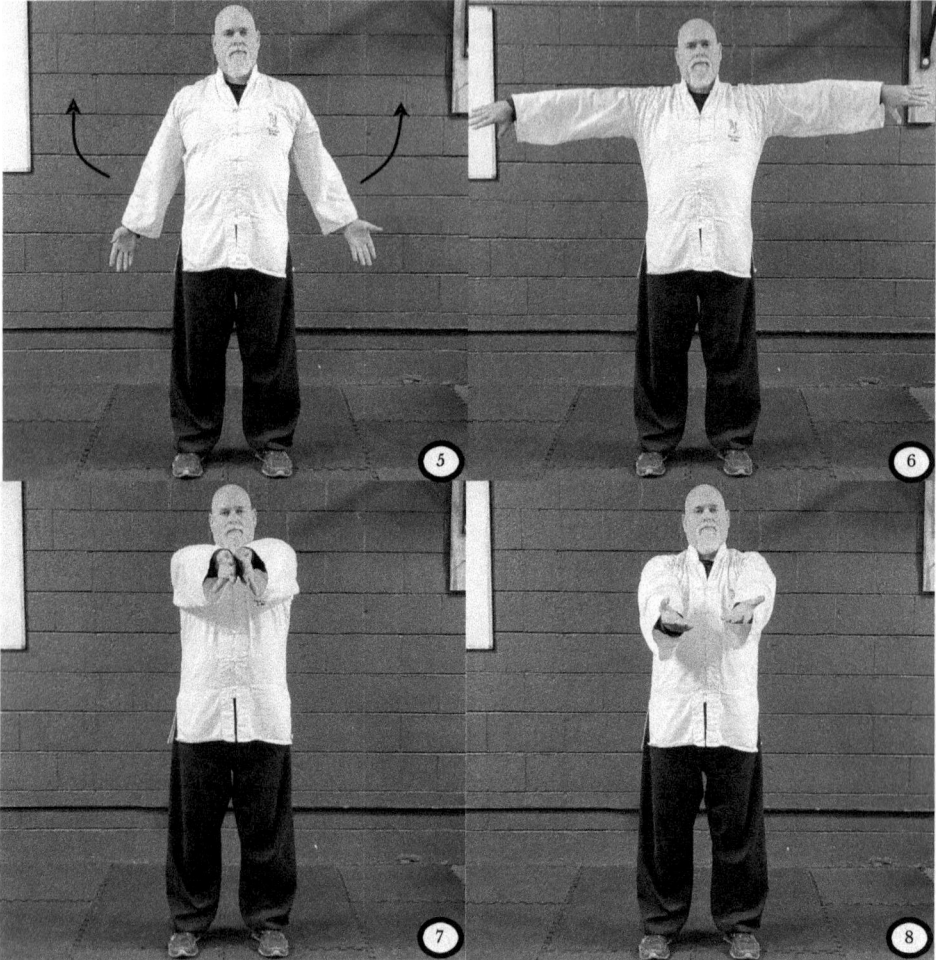

- **Elongation with spine turning.** 1. Hold a ball in the front of your abdomen. 2. Bring your hands up to your chest, palms up, with the fingers facing each other. 3-4. Separate hands and push one hand up and one hand down. 5. Turn to the right, the right hand goes palm up to the sky while the left hand goes palm down towards the ground.

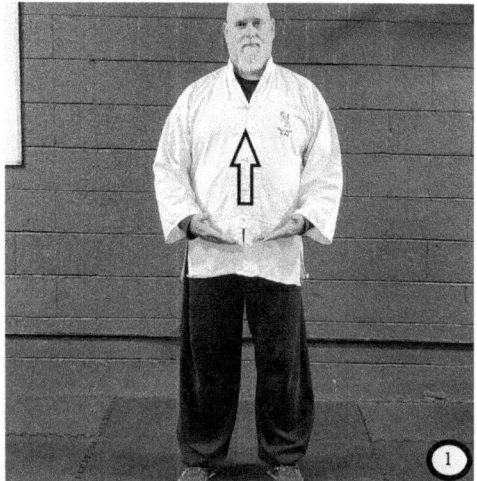

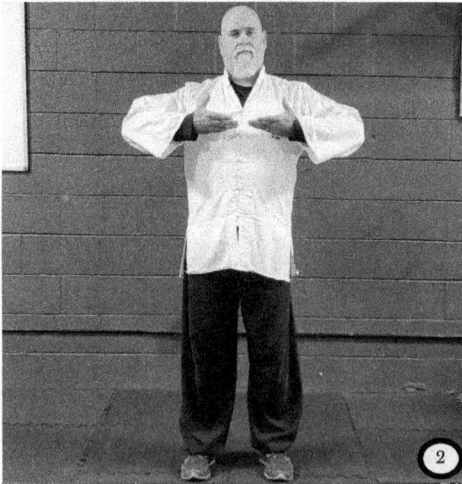

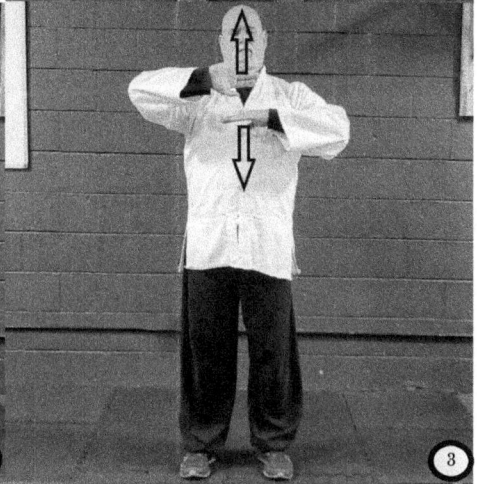

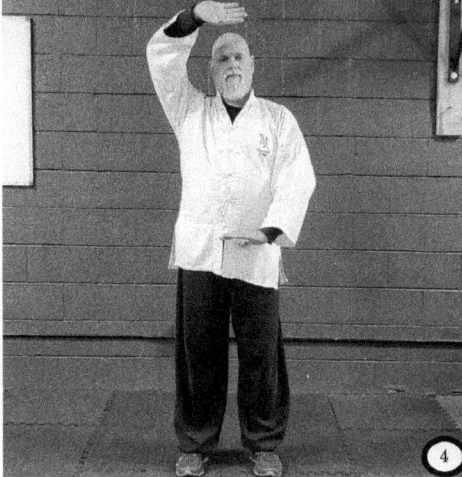

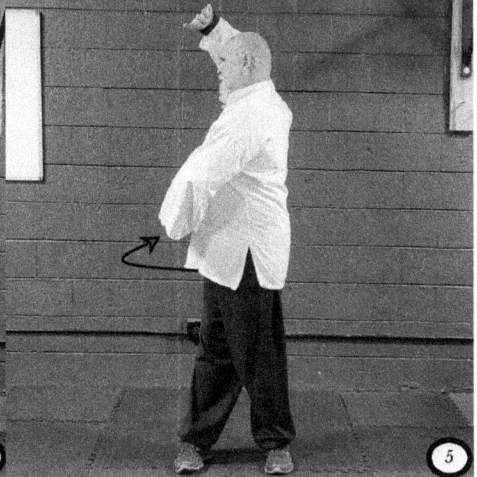

- **Elongation with spine turning**

6-10. Come back to the center and repeat on the left side. Don't lock your knees or hold your breath while performing this exercise. Keeps the spine healthy.

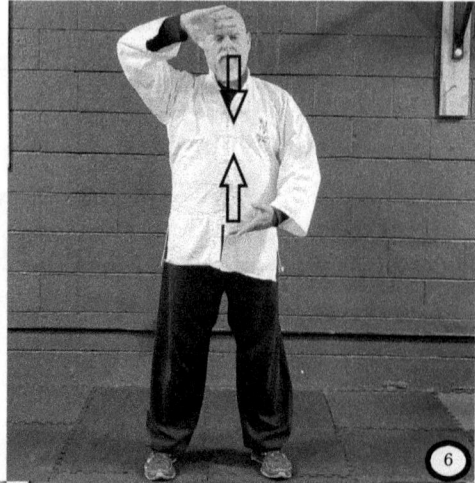

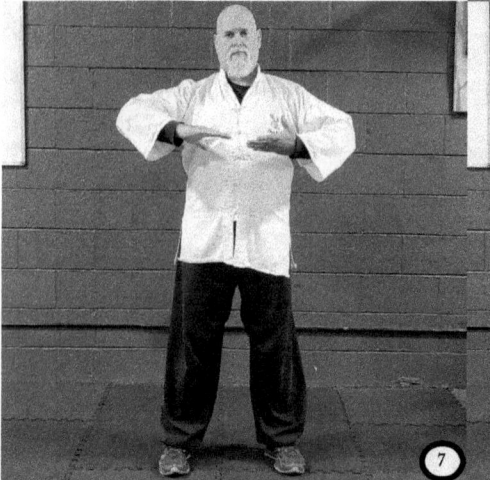

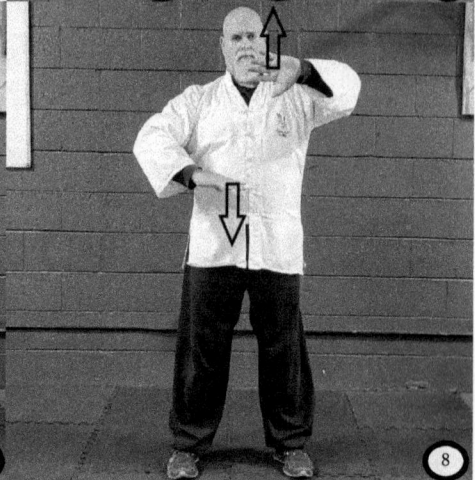

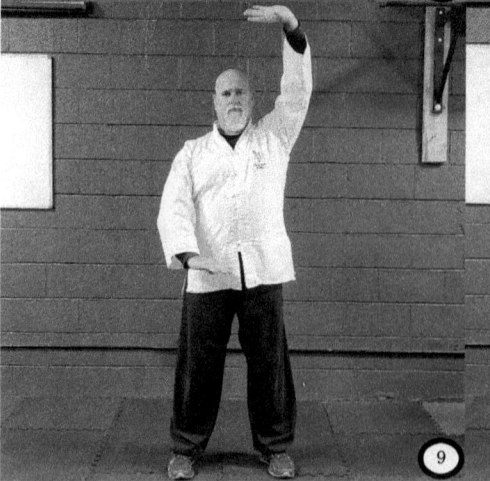

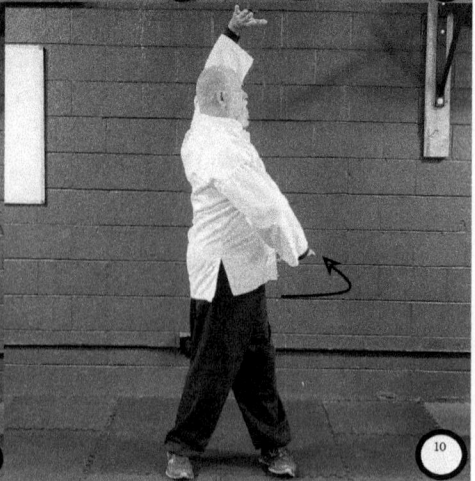

- **Elongation with spine turning while bending knees.** Same as above but add a squatting motion to each repetition when your hips face to the front.

- **Forward bend and stand. 1.** Start with your feet more than shoulder-width apart, don't lock your knees. **2.** Bend forward at the waist. **3-4.** Slowly come up one vertebra at a time. The last part of your body that comes up is your head.

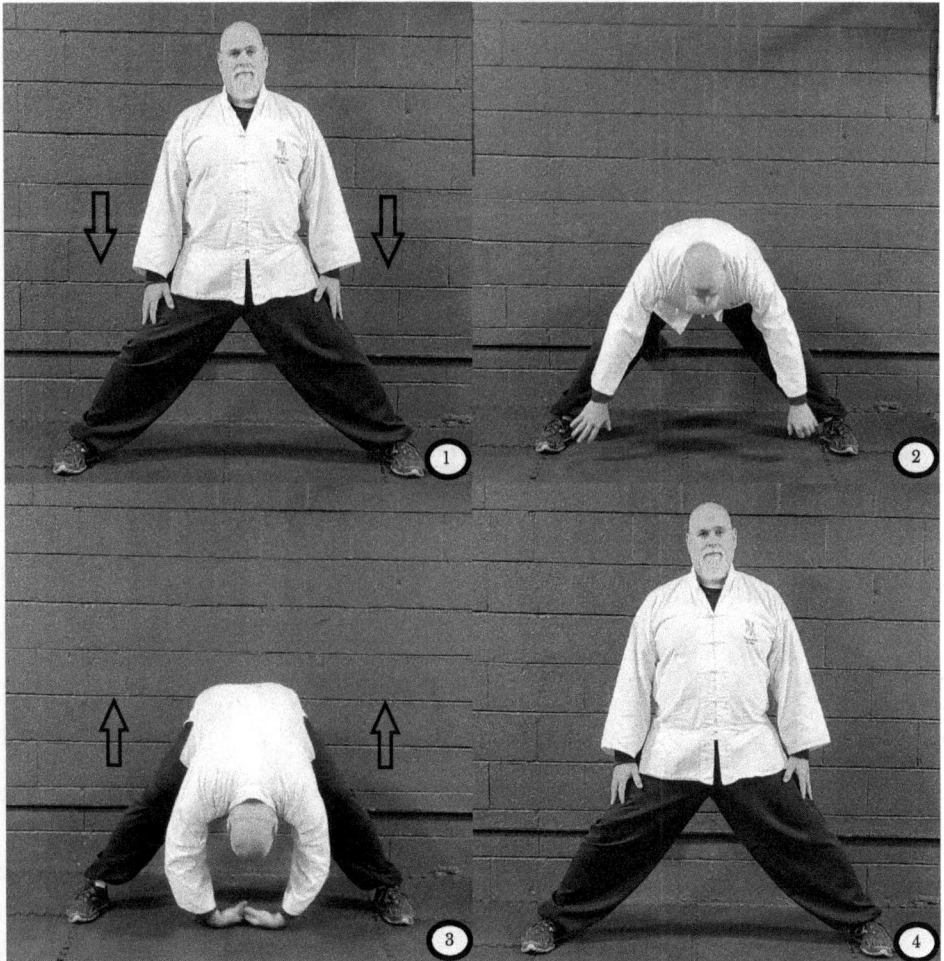

- **Neck stretch. 1.** Touch your chin to your chest. **2.** Move your head back to look at the ceiling. Bring your head back to the center. **3-4.** Move your head to the side bringing your ear closer to your shoulder, then repeat on the other side.

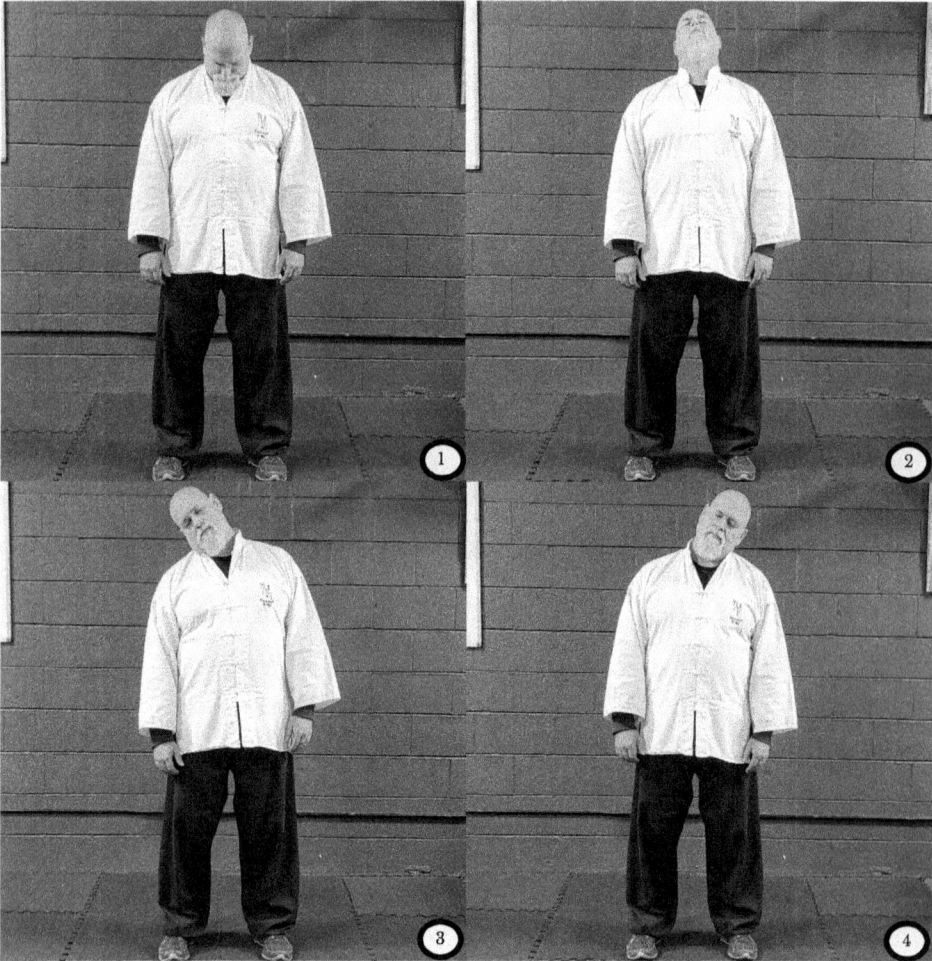

- **Pick the fruit off the tree.** 1. Feet are shoulder width apart. Raise your hands above your head, stretching fingers up. Reach up with your right hand, then bring it back down stopping just above the level of your shoulder. **2.** Then reach with your left hand. Repeat by alternating sides. Stretches the sides of the trunk. My teacher used to call this "mankind's oldest exercise".

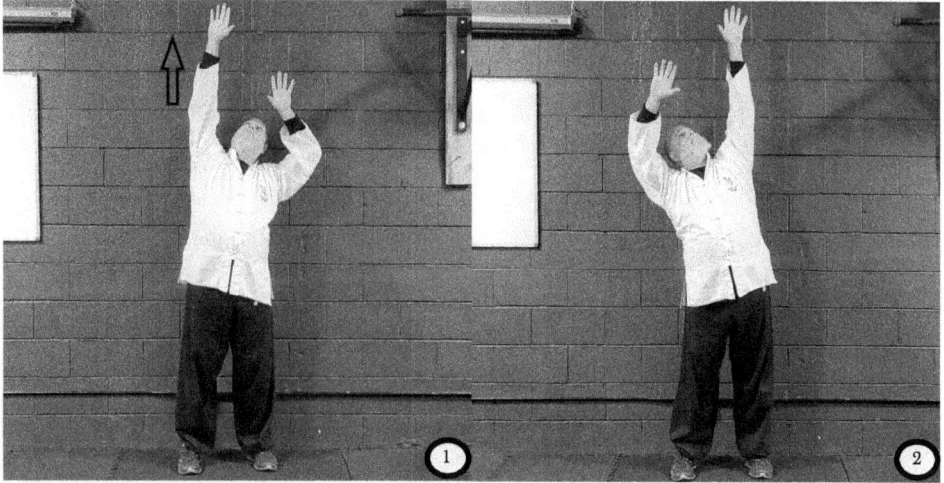

- **Shoulder circles**. 1. Begin exercise with your feet shoulder width apart. Bring arms are straight up over your head. 2. Bring your right hand backwards and let your torso turn to the right as you do so. 3. Turn left bringing your hips to the center, while continuing to make a circle with your arm, facing to the front with both arms down. 4. Continue turning to the left, your left arm circles up as your torso turns to the left. Let your waist turn back and forth naturally. Finish where you started.

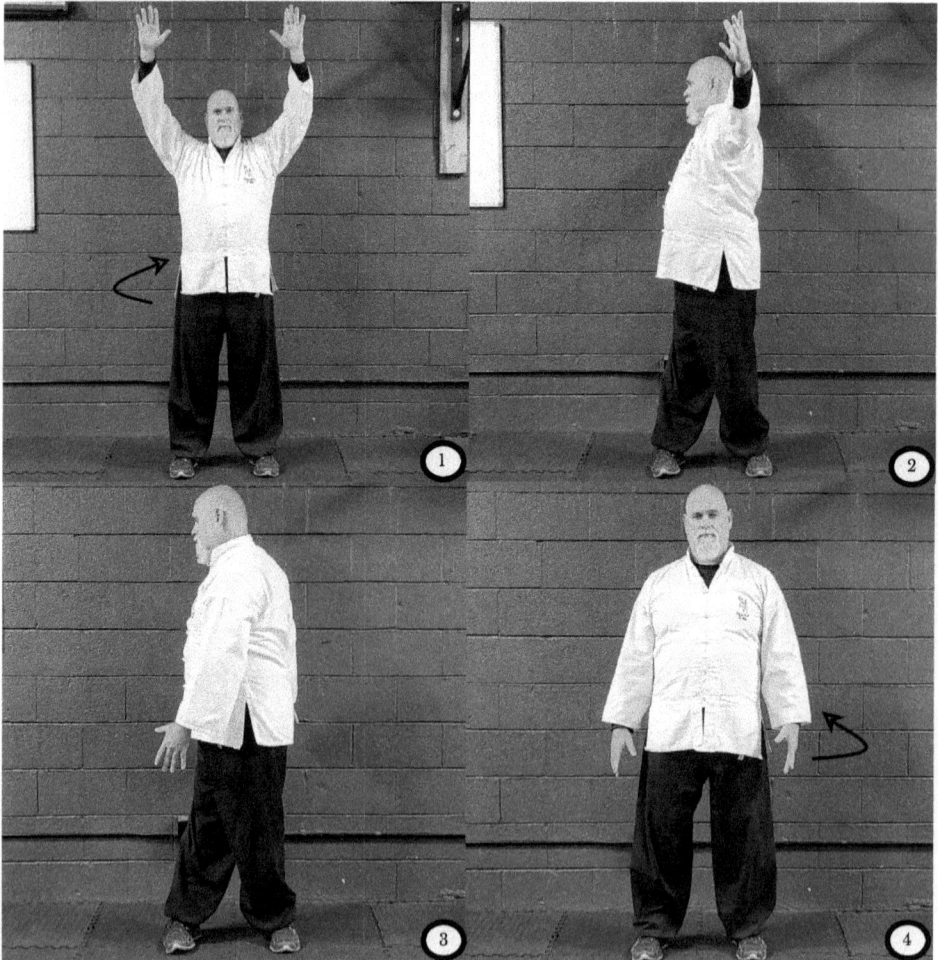

- **Shoulder stretch.** Bring one arm across your chest, then bend your other arm up cradling the arm that is across your chest by bending at the elbow. Pull the arm you are stretching into your chest to stretch the shoulder. Repeat on both sides.

Shoulder stretch (front view)   **Shoulder stretch (side view)**

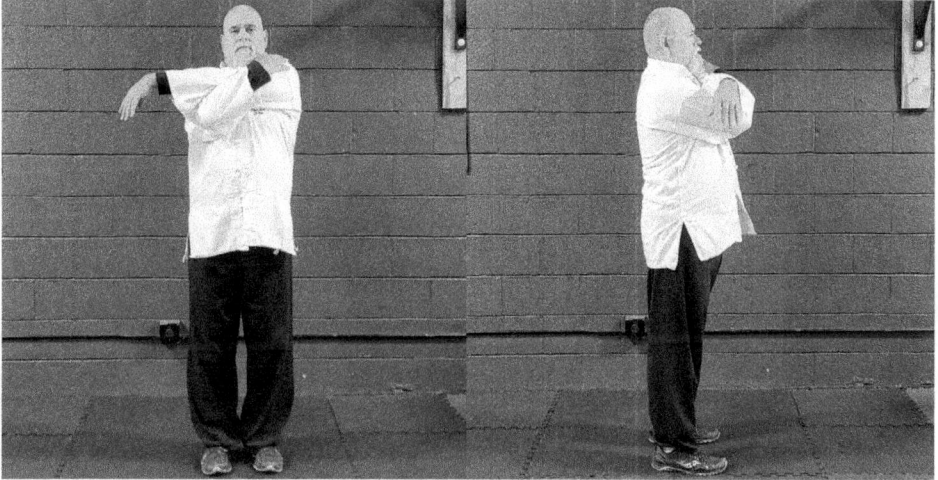

- **Upper back stretch.** Feet are shoulder width apart. Interlock your fingers, rotate your palms out, and stretch your arms forward, arms parallel to the ground.

Upper back stretch (front view)   **Upper back stretch (side view)**

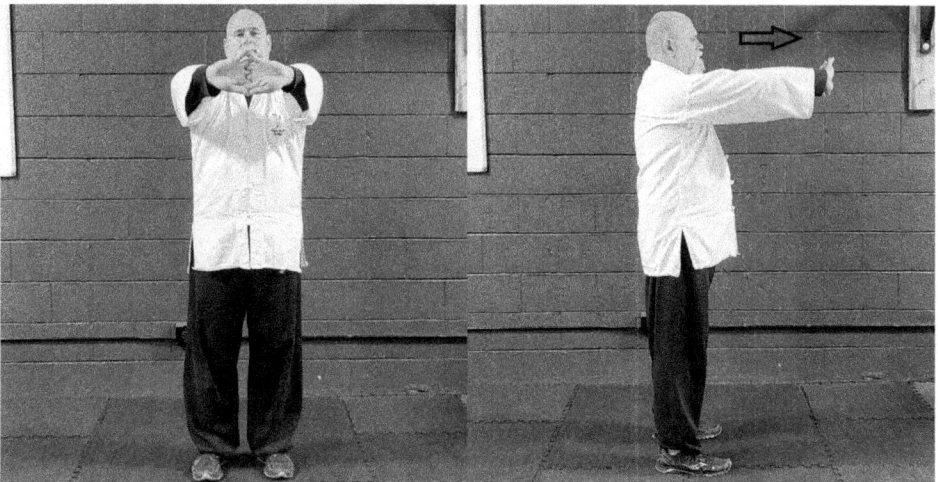

- **Standing groin stretch.** Bring your feet about twice shoulder width apart, and bend one leg, hold for 10-30 seconds. Switch to the other side. Hold for 10-30 seconds then slowly return to standing position. It is not necessary fully bend your knee to perform this exercise. Don't bend so far forward that this exercise strains your back.

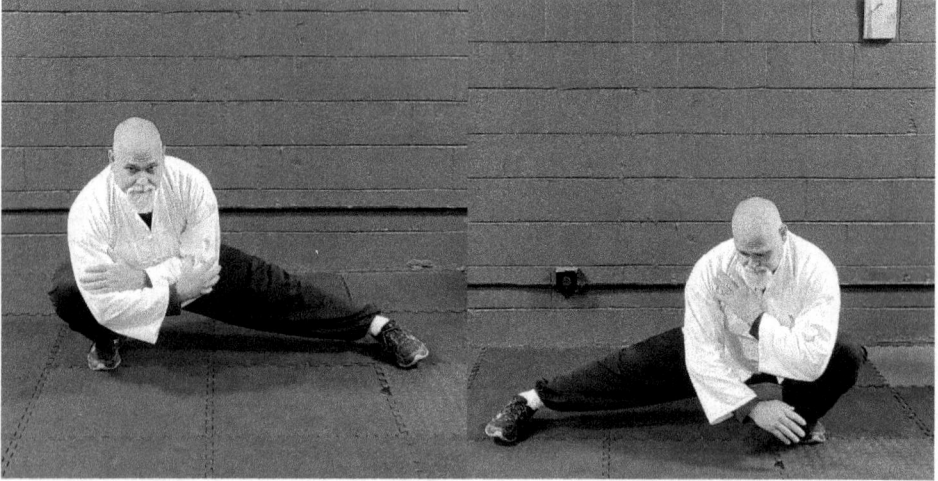

- **Wrist stretches** (outer, downward, inward). **Outer:** Place the thumb of one hand on the back of your other hand while simultaneously grabbing the base of the thumb with your fingers. Push with your thumb while pulling with your fingers turning the wrist joint out. **Downward:** Grab the back of one hand with the palm of the other and push the wrist joint down. **Inward:** Place the palms of both hands together and push.

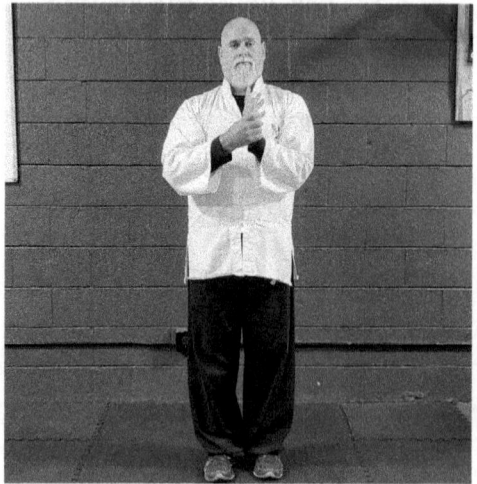

Outer wrist stretch

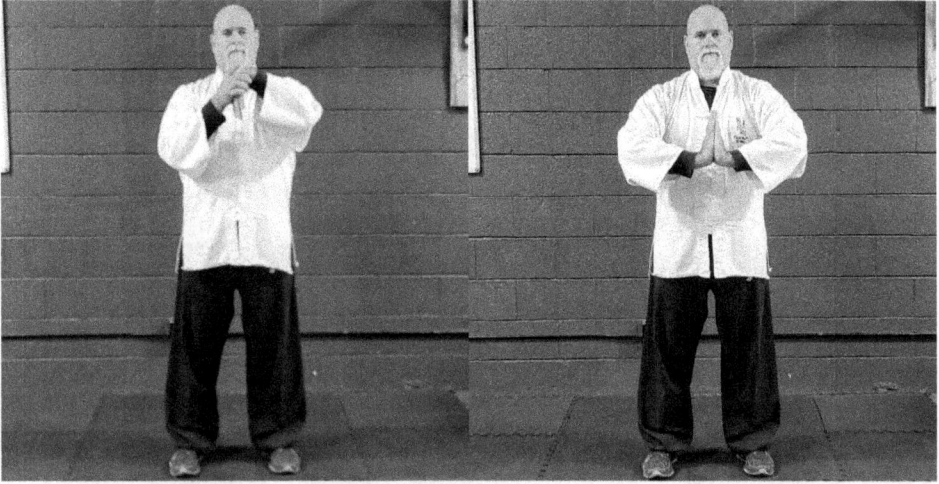

Downward wrist stretch   Inward wrist stretch

Warm-Up Exercises

Warm-up exercises are done for 10-15 minutes after rotations and stretching. Do not force the warm-up exercises. None of the following exercises should hurt; if they do don't do them. These exercises should not be done to the point that they induce sweating. Don't hold your breath or lock your knees while performing these exercises.

Each exercise is intended to support one or more aspects of tai chi. Breath, rooting, relaxation, posture, structure, and *qi* circulation are examples. The warm-up exercises also improve a student's strength and balance, and support overall health.

- **Alternating crane stances. 1.** Shift your weight to the left leg and turn the left foot out 45 degrees. Lift the right leg above the waist, bent at the knee, and hold for 10 seconds, and return to the ground with control. **2.** Switch to the other leg. Improves balance and leg strength.

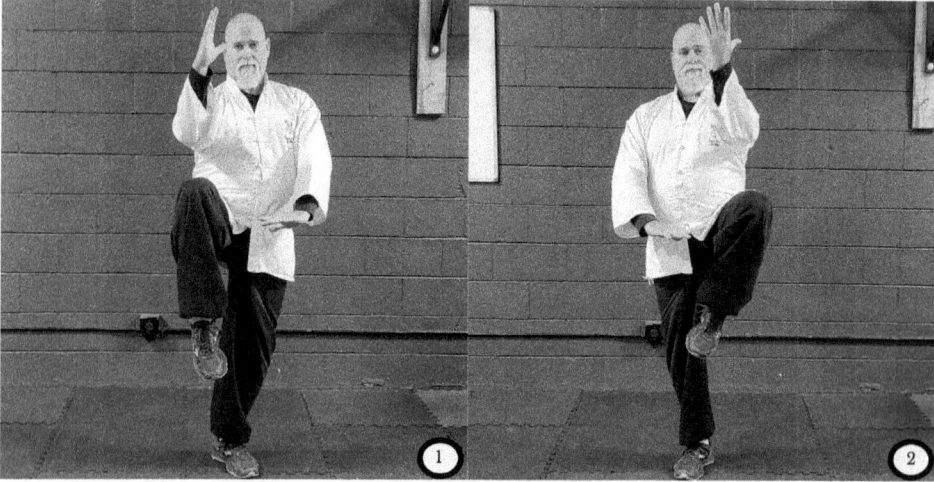

- **Calf raises. 1.** Start with feet shoulder width apart. **2.** Lift your body up onto your toes and hold for 3-5 seconds. Return heels to the ground and repeat. You can hold onto a chair or a wall to help with balance.

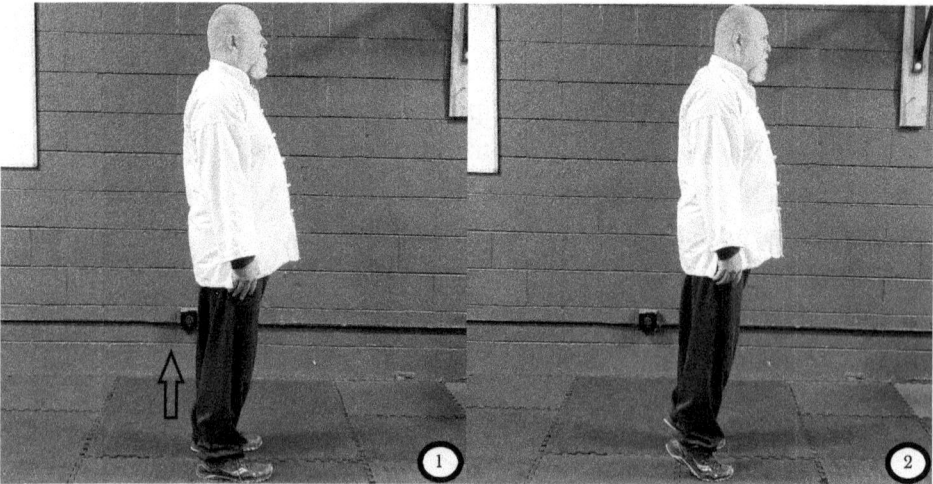

- **Embracing the tree.** Static training, try to hold for 3-5 minutes. This can be done from either the small horse stance or the traditional horse stance. Arms are held in front of your body, palms facing in like you are holding a large ball. Elbows are soft and bent slightly. Palms face in. Push your head towards the ceiling. Relax your upper back, shoulders, and jaw. Make your hips level and parallel with the ground. This is an excellent exercise for inducing the *qi* sensation in the arms and is frequently used during qi gong practice.

Embracing the Tree (side view)   Embracing the Tree (front view)

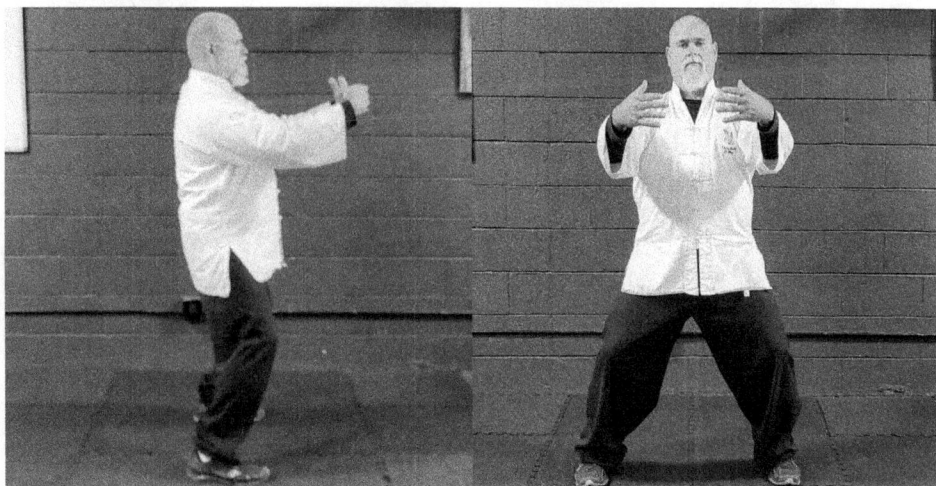

- **Commence tai chi. 1.** Sink your *qi* into the ground and practice rooting. **2.** Move your arms forward and up until they are parallel to the ground. **3.** Move the back of the hands towards the chest with the fingers facing forward and the palms flat. **4.** Push palms down. Elbows are soft and pointing down. Sink your weight by slightly bending your knees. Inhale as your arms go up and exhale as your arms go down.

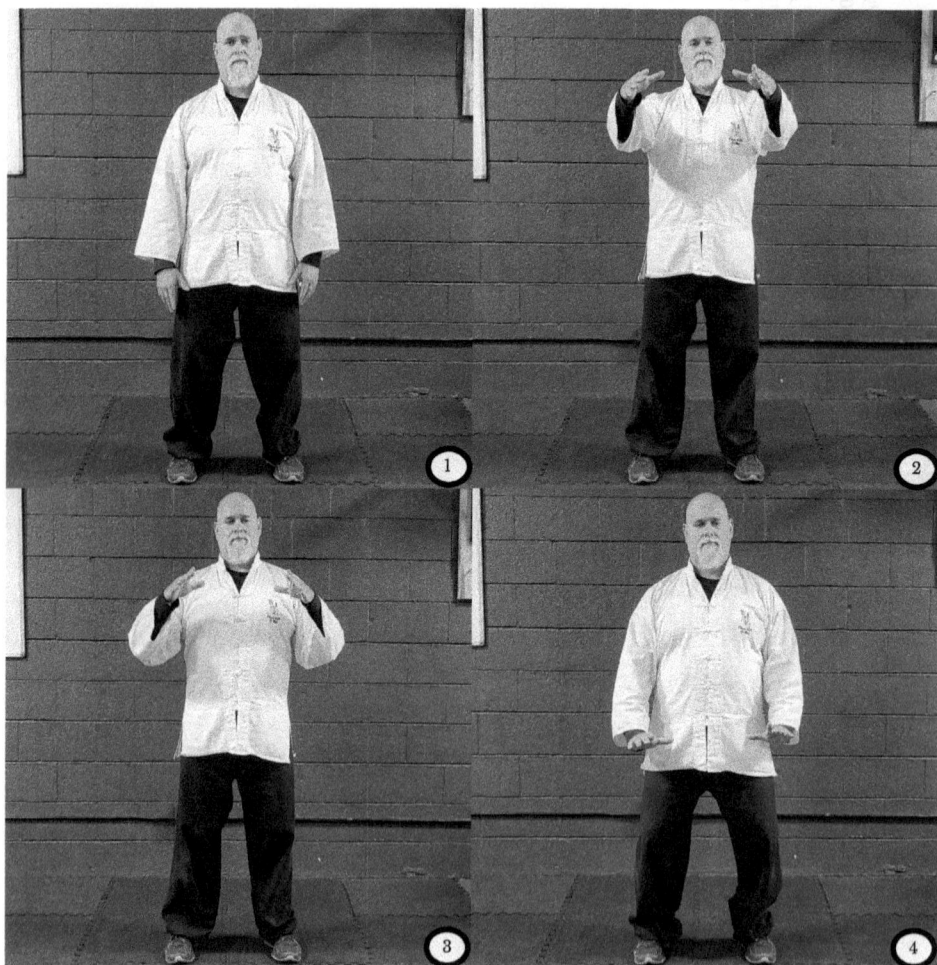

Commence tai chi (side view)

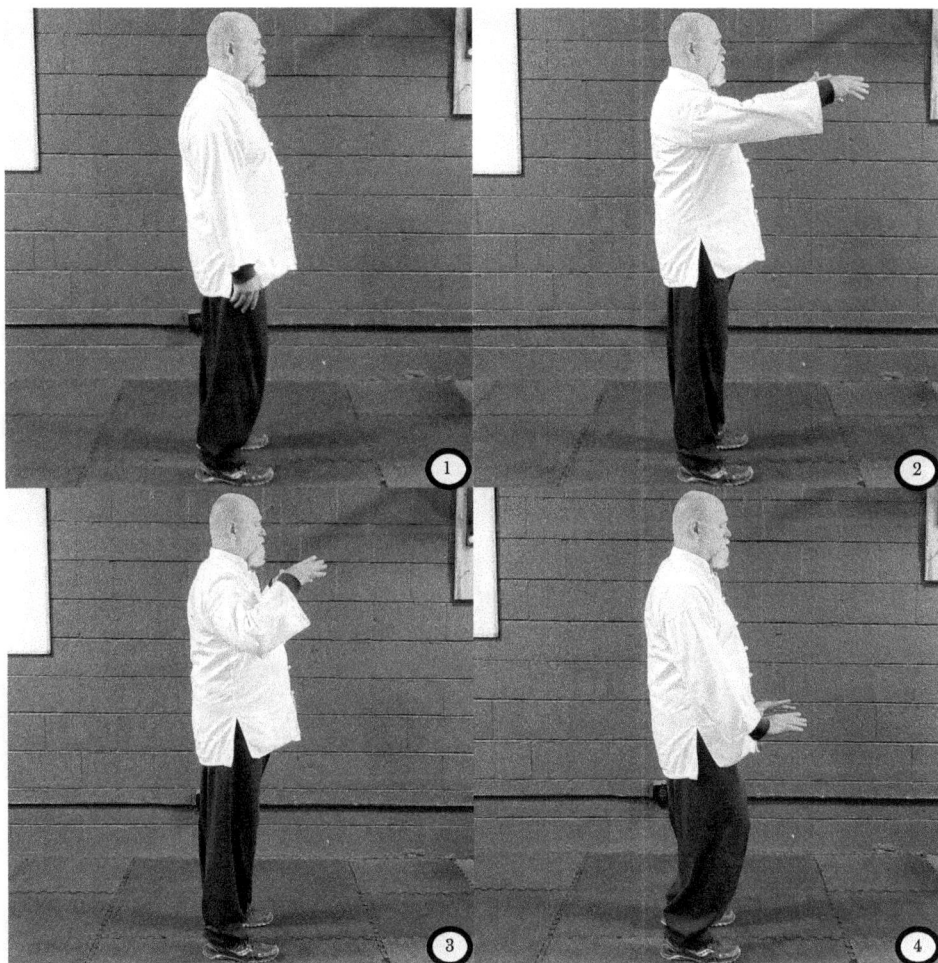

- **Opening the spine.** This is a fairly advanced exercise. Flex and extend the spine. **1.** Start with the palms of the hands together. **2.** As you bend forward and flex your spine, your elbows should move closer together. As you return to the starting position (spinal extension) your elbows should move apart. Avoid using your arm or shoulder muscles. Keeping your spine mobile and flexible will improve your health. In TCM we say, "You are only as old as your spine."

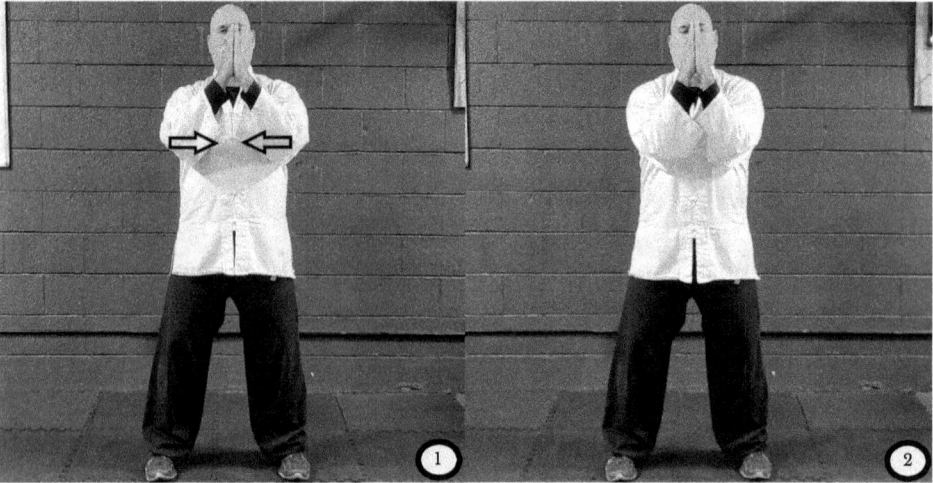

- **Polishing the mirror. 1.** Keep the back straight and the head up. **2.** Bend at the knees, hands are facing to the front, palms face out. As you bend your knees hands move down and then out. **3-5.** As you straighten your legs the hands move up. Repeat. Leg and low back strengthening exercise.

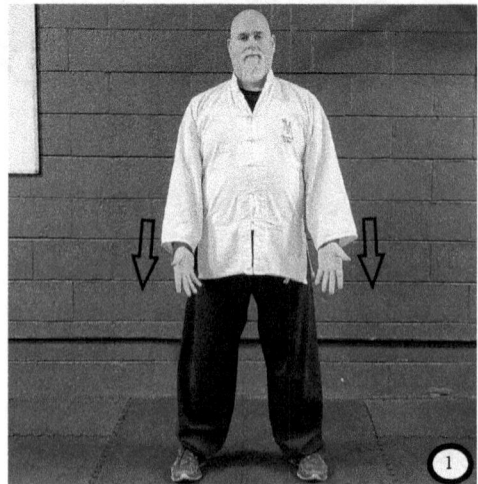

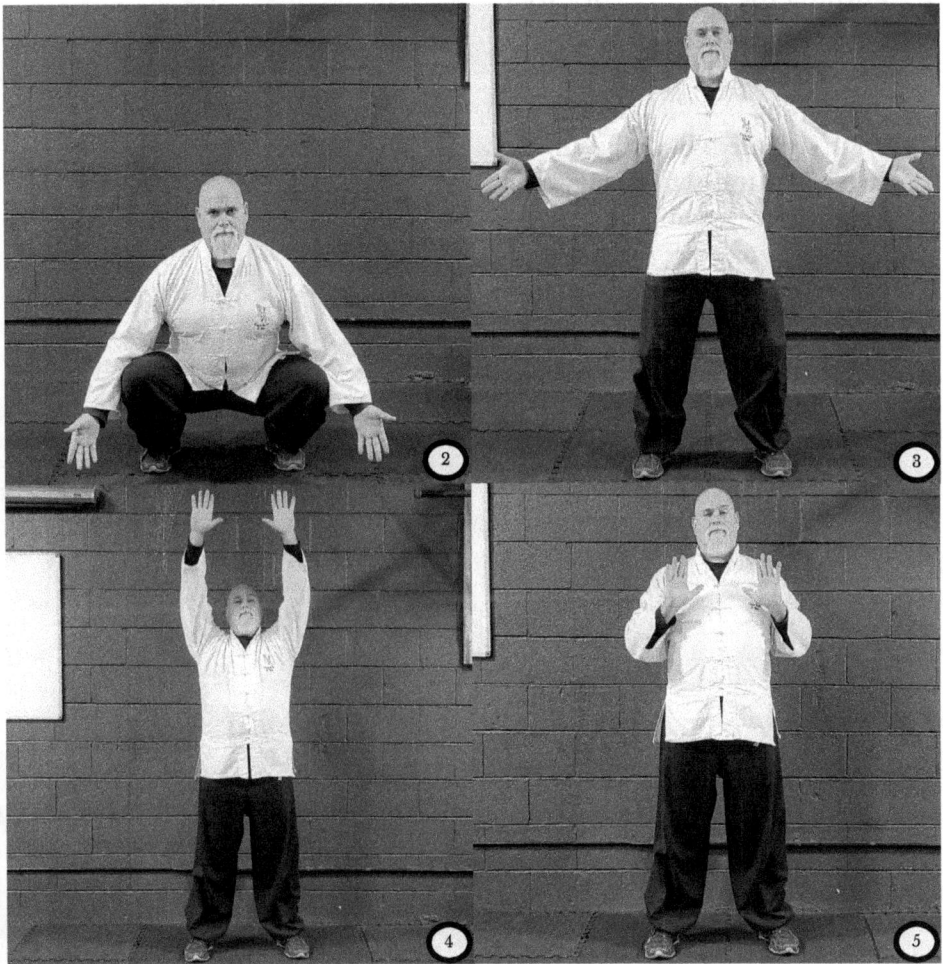

- **Pushing the wall.** Weight transferring exercise. Practice making smooth transitions from right to left. Pay close attention to proper knee/foot alignment. Avoid bending your knees laterally as you move to the side. This exercise teaches you how to shift your weight by turning your hip and bending your knee. 1. Start with feet shoulder width apart.

- **Pushing the wall. 2**. Turn to left keeping your feet facing forward. Shift your weight to the left leg by pushing off with your right leg. **3**. Let your hips swing naturally to the right. **4**. Leading with your *tan tien*, push off your left leg bringing your torso to the right, weight transfers to the right leg. **5**. Turn your torso to the left, push off your right leg shifting your weight to the left and re-peat on the right side.

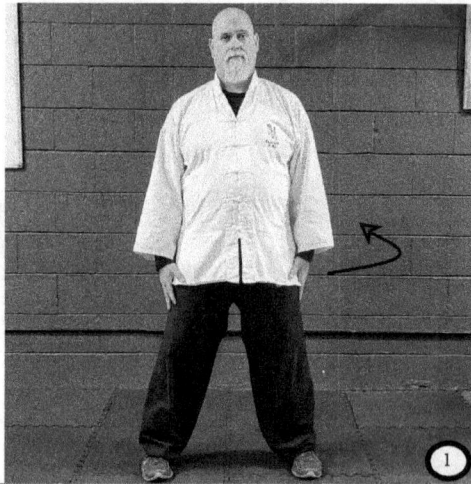

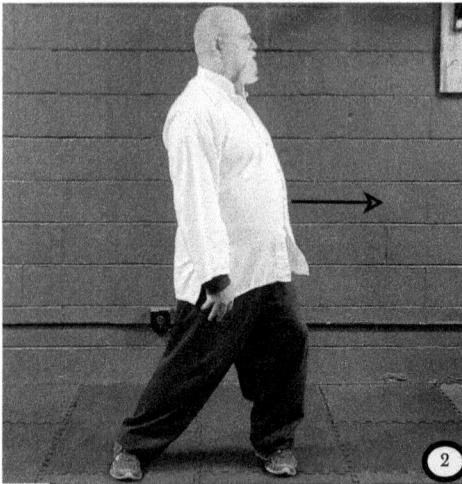

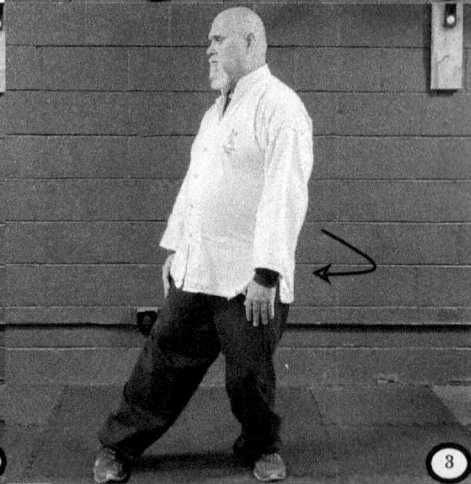

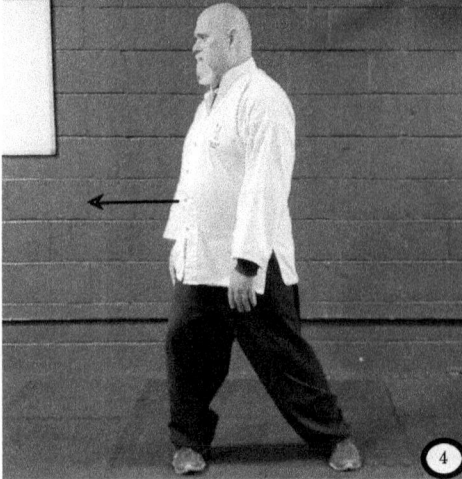

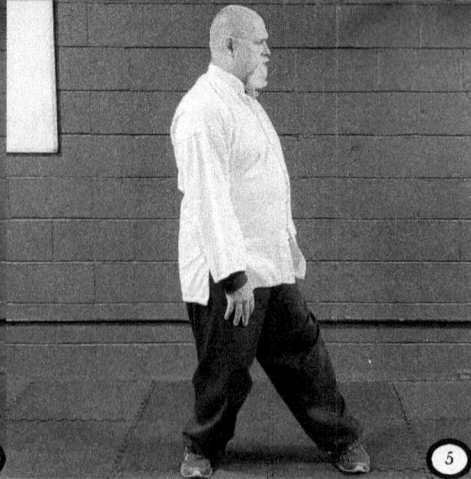

- **Scooping the air.** 1. Starting from a horse stance. **2.** Squat and bring both hands in and down like making a scooping motion. **3-4.** Straighten your legs, lift arms up. Repeat. For an extra level of difficulty go into a calf raise as you come up to the standing position. Lower body strengthening exercise.

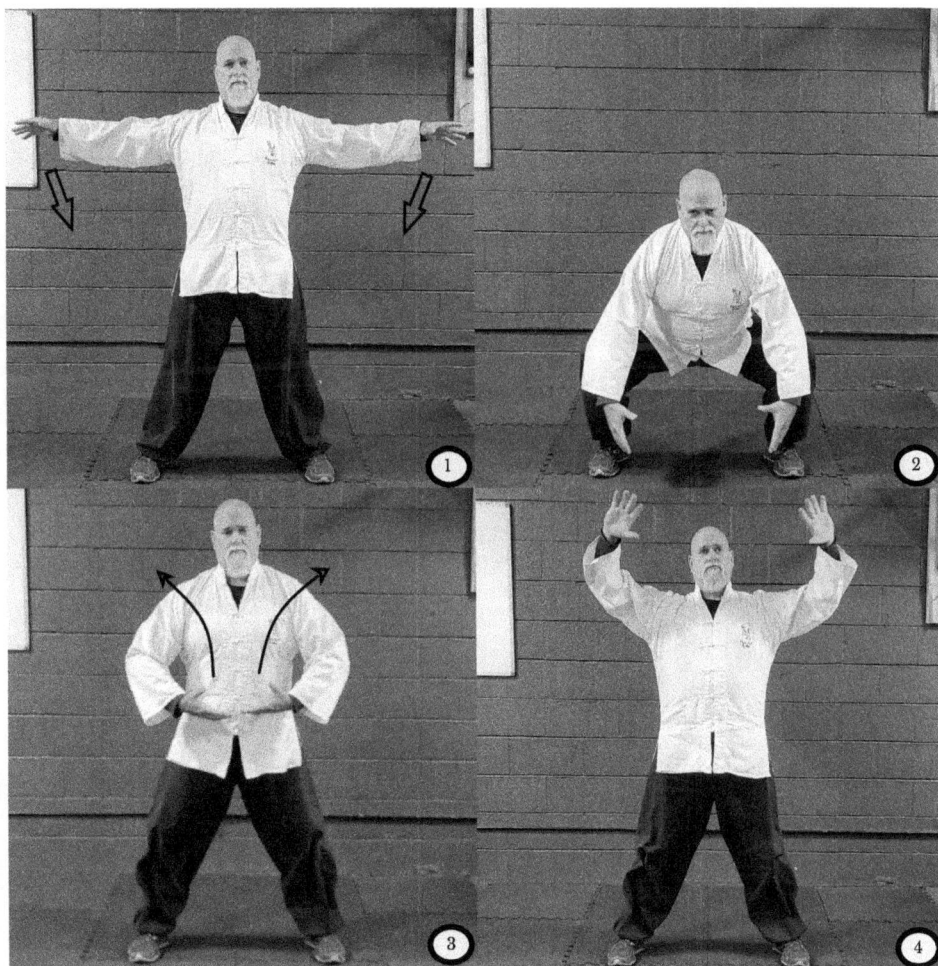

- **Shifting ball.** Your lower body is in a traditional horse stance. **1.** Your hands start off in the hold right ball posture. **2.** Shift your ball forward, bringing your hands to the front of your chest. **3.** Then move the ball to the left, ending in the hold left ball posture. Turn from the waist and keep your elbows pointing down. Feet stay firmly planted throughout.

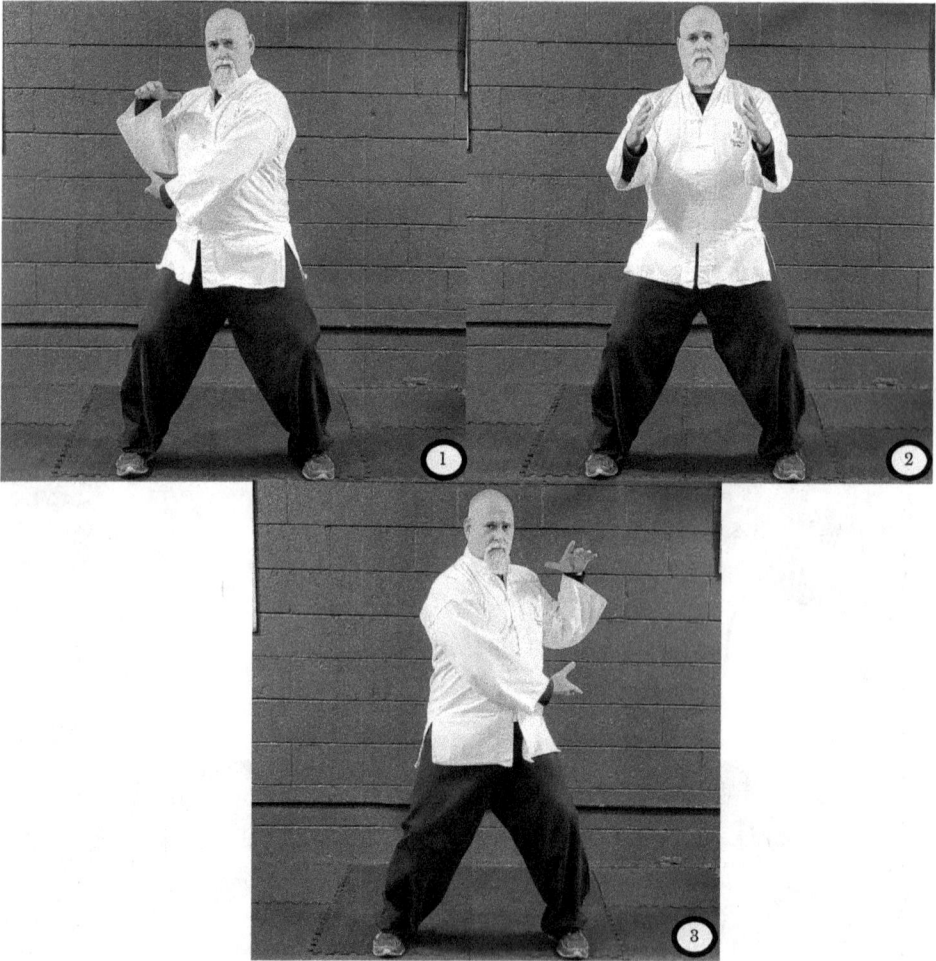

- **Static stance training.** Move into one of these stances and hold: traditional or small horse stance, cat stance, crane stance, 60/40 stance. Alternate as needed. These stances will improve lower body strength and balance.

- **Square horse/*tan tien* breathing.** Square horse is practiced to strengthen the lower body and legs. Hold this posture, relax body, and breathe into the *tan tien*. Visualize *qi* flowing into the ground through your feet.

- **Shifting bow stance exercise. 1.** Start out in a 60/40 stance. **2-3.** Practice shifting the weight from front to back. When your weight is shifted forward your hips point in the same direction as your lead foot. When your weight is shifted over your back foot, your hips turn to face the same direction as your back foot. Don't bend forward at the waist.

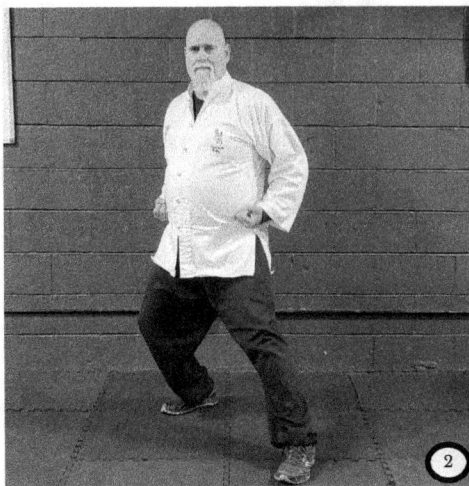

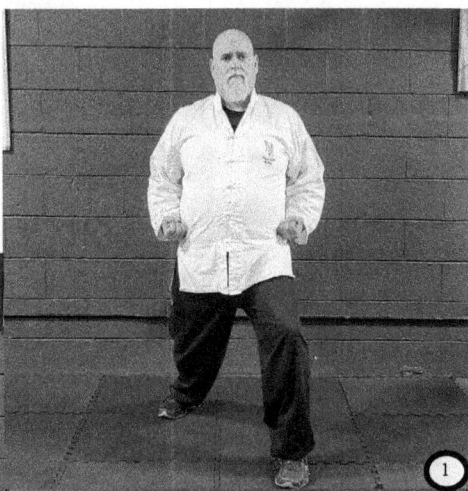

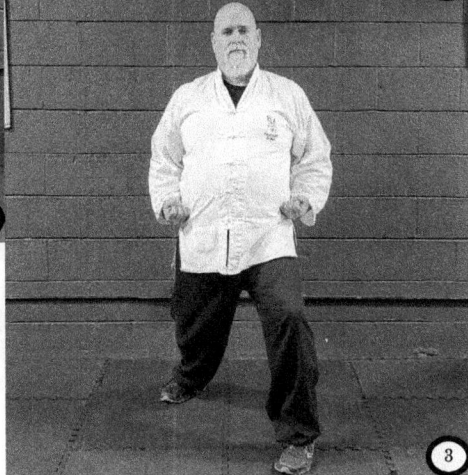

- **Turn and slap palms. 1.** Start with feet a little more than shoulder width apart. During this exercise, keep your feet stationary. **2.** Using your core muscles, turn your waist to the right, forcing your hands to slap together on the right side. Look at the hands that are slapping. **3-4.** Alternate sides. Avoid using your arm muscles to move your hands together, instead use the momentum from the waist turning. Puts the spine into torsion. Also helps strengthen *tan tien*/core muscles.

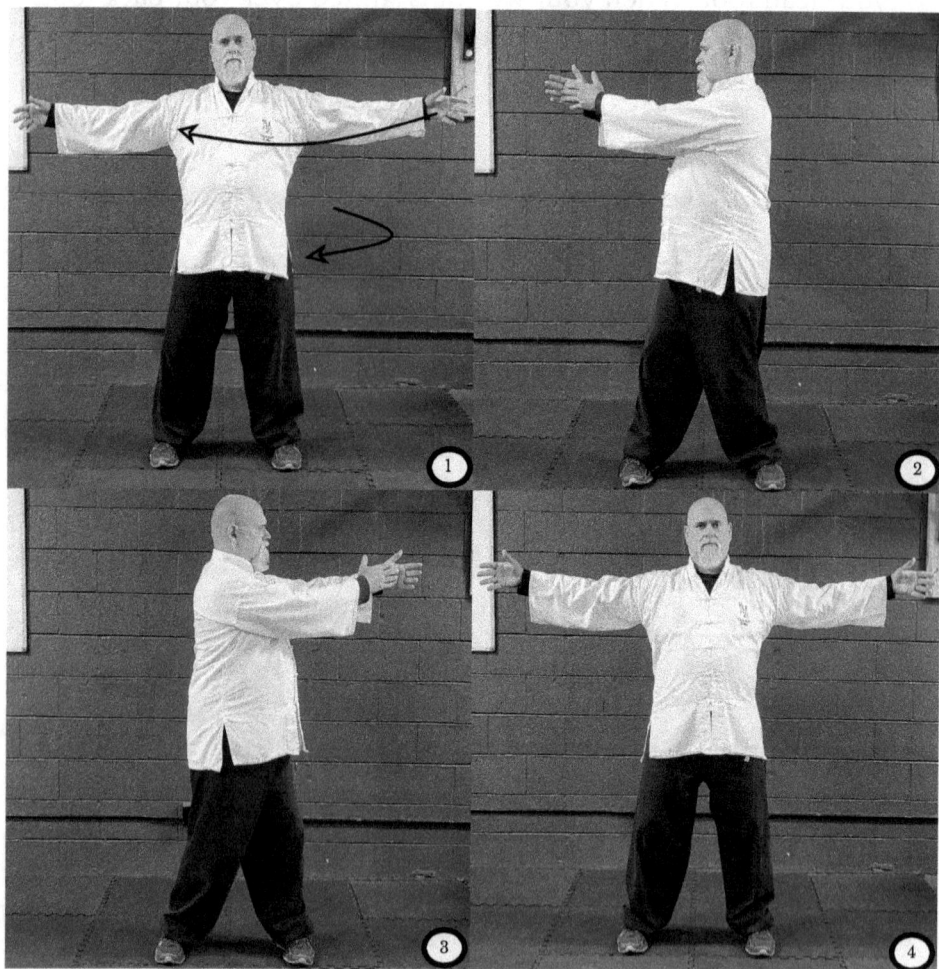

- **Turn trunk and gaze at moon. 1.** Start by holding a ball in front of the *tan tien*. Keeping your feet stationary, slowly turn your trunk and waist to the left. **2.** When you turn to the left your left arm leads and is higher than the right arm. Eyes look at the hand that is higher. You should feel torsion in your spine. Hold for 3-5 seconds. Repeat on both sides.

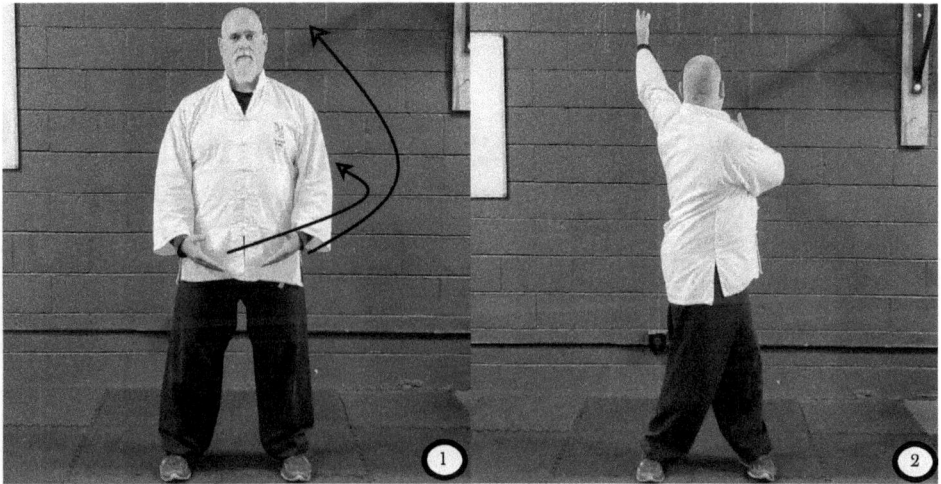

- **Waist turning.** Start in the small horse stance. Both hands in front of you like they are resting on a table. Release any tension in your shoulders and upper back. Practice turning your waist left and right without engaging your hips or legs. Keep arms in position. Then practice turning your torso using only your hip joints. This exercise is good for helping to discern the difference between movement at the hips versus movement at the waist. It can also help identify abdominal and core muscles.

- **Waist turning with arms hitting.** Start with feet slightly more than shoulder width apart. For this exercise, keep your feet stationary. 1. Turn the waist and hips to the left. 2. Let your arms strike your torso with a loose fist or open hand on the front and back. **3-6.** Turn torso to the right and repeat, alternating to both sides. The skill here is to learn how to guide force into your arms from the ground without using your arm muscles, and still get them to move. You want to feel the vibration from the hits to your torso.

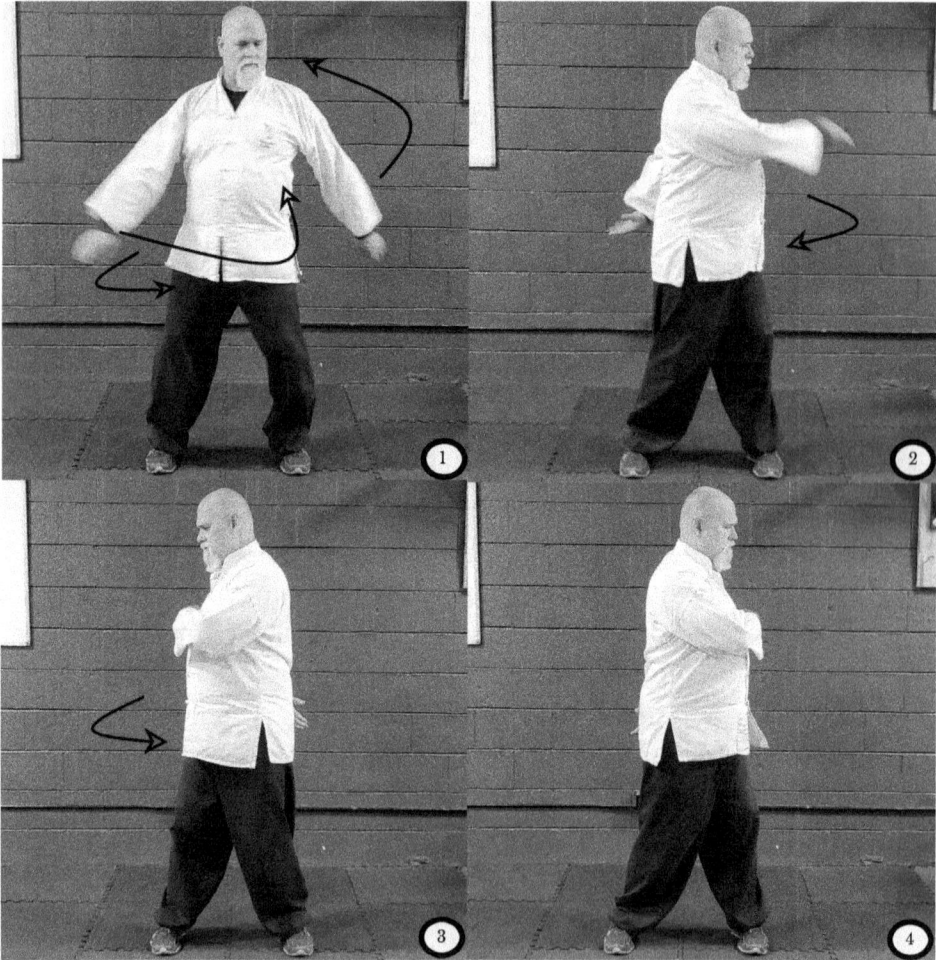

- **Waist turning with arms hitting**

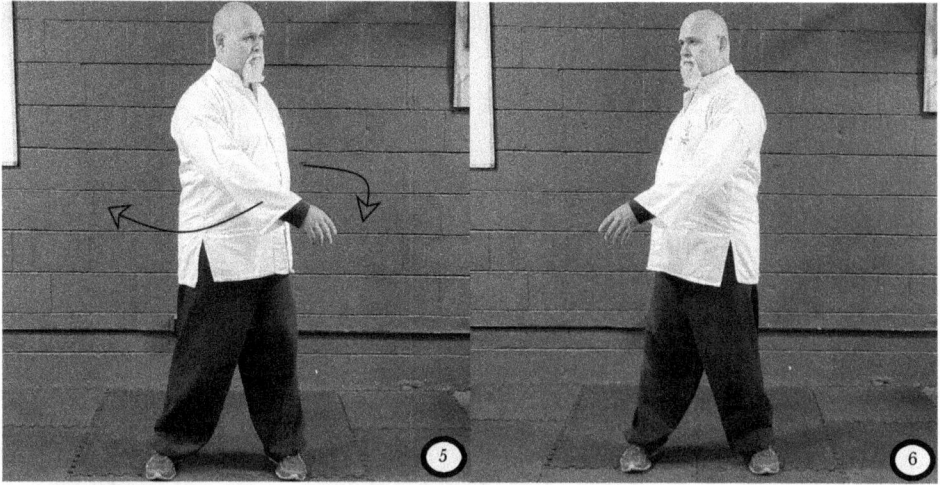

- **Waist turning with arms hitting (variation).** Same set up and general motions as the previous exercise but guide your hands to the top of your shoulders/traps. You can incorporate flexion and extension at the knees, straightening your legs as your hand move up to strike your traps.

- **Wardoff.** 1. From a cat stance, holding a right ball. **2.** Step forward into a 60/40 stance with your left foot and wardoff with your left arm. **3-4.** Same movement viewed from the side. At the same time bring your right hand, palm down, fingers forward, to your right hip, just in front of the hip flexors. Rock back, taking the weight off your left foot and lift the left toes. Rotate the left foot out, step up with right foot into a cat stance. Repeat on the right side.

Wardoff (front view)

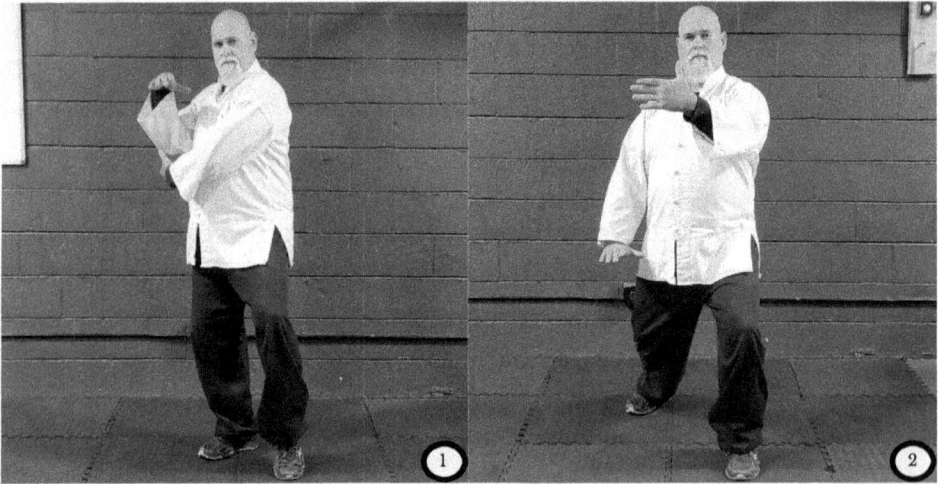

Wardoff (side view)

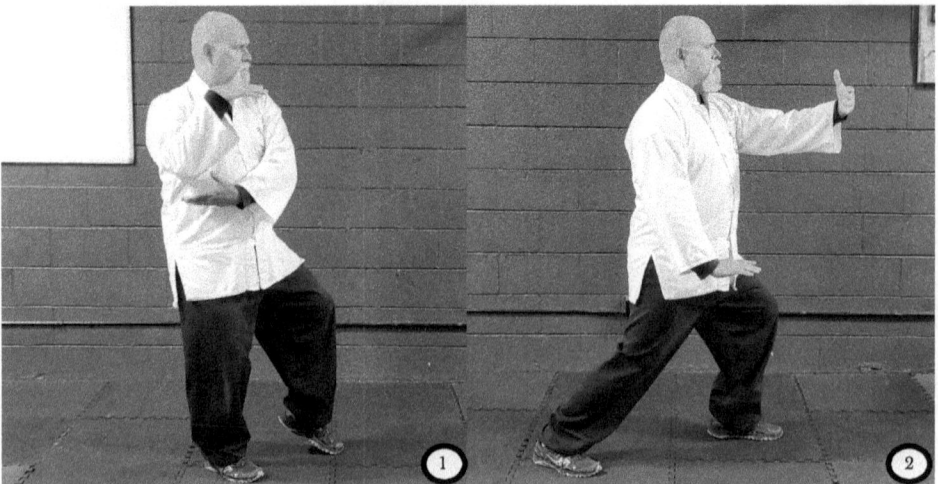

- **Wave hands like clouds.** Practice this technique in the same way you perform it in the empty hand form, but your feet remain stationary. Throughout this exercise your arms move left to right through the motion of the spine and not with your arm muscles. When your hands go down let gravity do the work. When your hand move upwards use momentum. Practice directing your arms through the motion of your hips and waist. 1. Start with feet shoulder width apart. Your right arm is held at chest level, your left hand is in front of your *tan tien*. 2. Hips turn to the right. Your right hand circles outward to the right, your left hand circles upwards to the right.

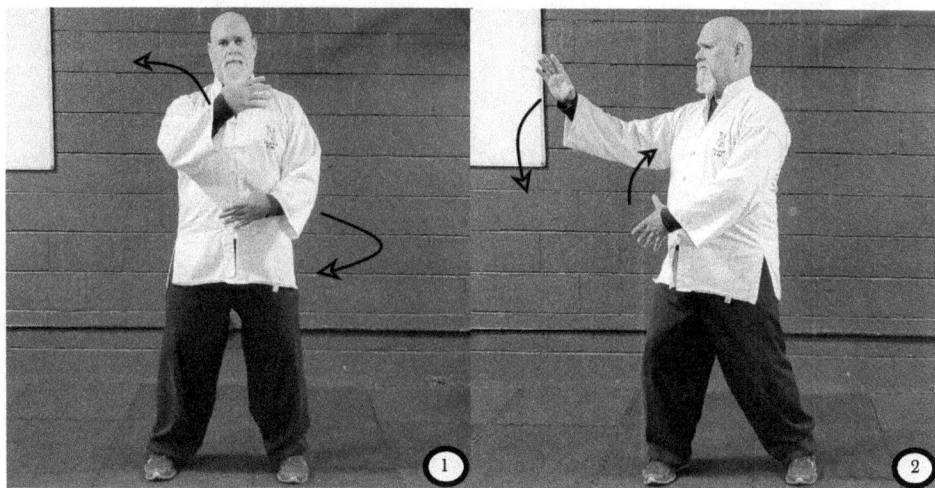

Wave hands like clouds. 3. Turn your hips to the left. **4.** Your hands move to the front of your torso, your left hand is at chest level and your right hand is at the level of your *tan tien*. **5.** Repeat on the left side.

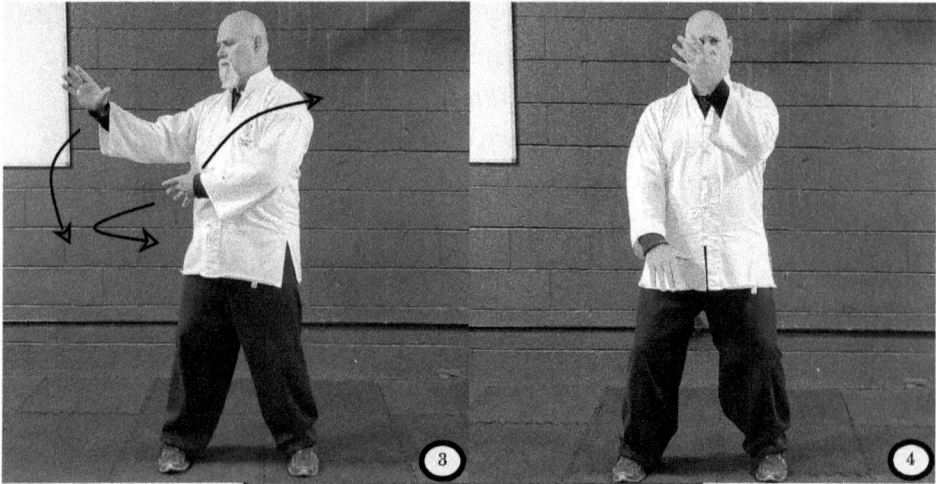

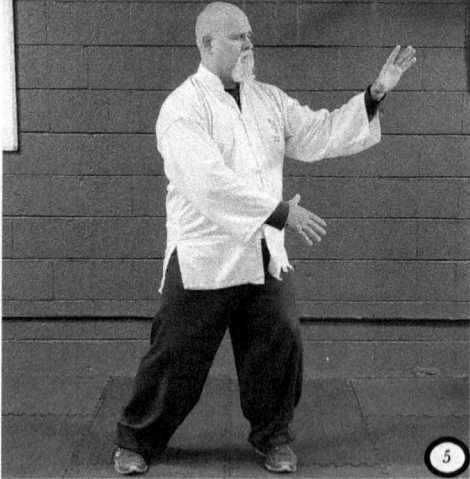

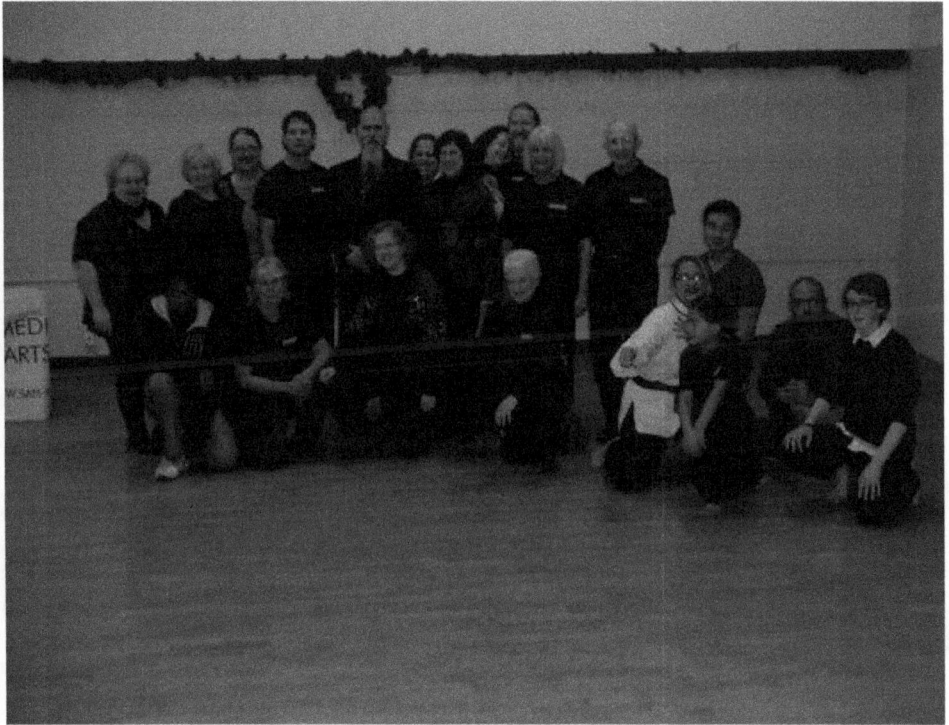

Students posing after performing at the
SAMMA End of Year Banquet in 2015

Tai Chi Basics

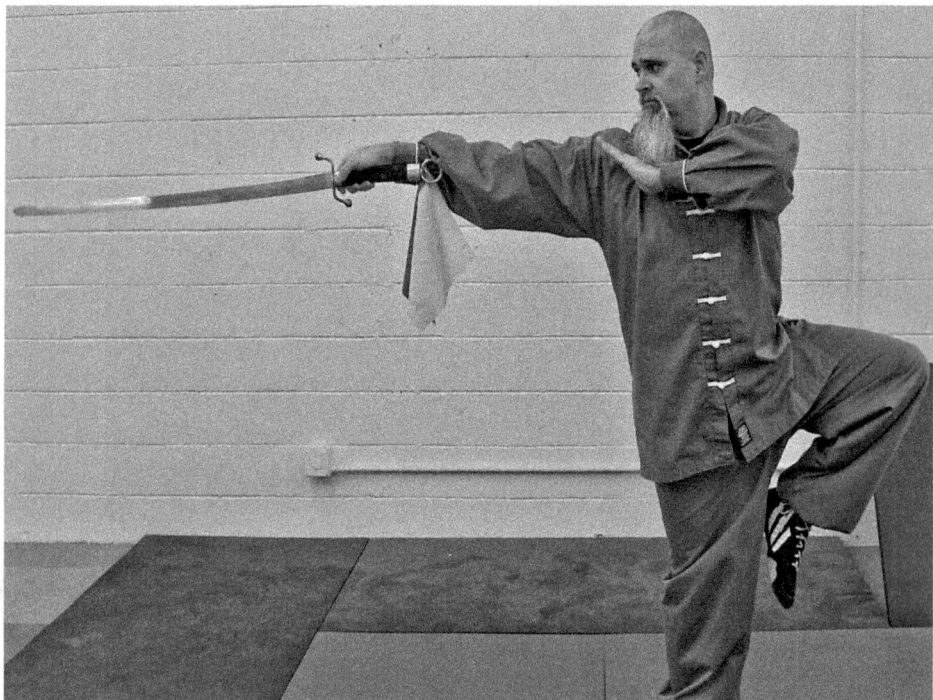

Tai Chi Saber

Stances

Stances can be thought of as temporary body structures that are adopted to confer some kind of martial advantage or to facilitate the execution of a technique. It is helpful to study and practice the correct weight distribution for each, to understand what each stance facilitates, and to use them in context of the movements they support. Each comes with built-in advantages and disadvantages, and each stance creates a line of stability and a line of instability.

If you imagine drawing a straight line that extends through the middle of each foot, this line becomes the line of stability, meaning that you have the strongest root when facing an attack from that direction. Drawing another imaginary line offset at a 90-degree angle will give you the line of instability, where you have the least balance and root.

Stances will generally attempt to turn your centerline away from your opponent's frontal attack. Your hands should always be doing one of three things—chambering, guarding, or executing a technique. Chambering refers to the placement of your hands, often at the waist, in preparation for a strike. Guarding is the positioning of your hands to protect your head, face, chest or groin. The hands can be open or closed in a fist, dictated by what you plan on doing with them.

- **Attention.** The feet are together, knees are slightly bent, weight is 50/50. Drop the tension out of your shoulders and push your head up to elongate the spine. Relax your shoulders and upper back to make the chest very slightly concave. Don't pluck out the chest. We start and end forms from the position of attention.

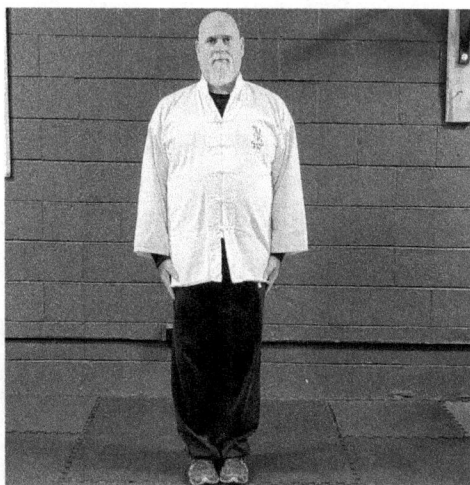

81

- **Cat stance** (heel up, heel down). A defensive stance with your back leg rooted and both knees bent. 90 percent of your weight is on your back leg, 10 percent on your front leg. Back should be generally straight with the head held erect. Don't let your head move past the imaginary vertical line created by your heels. The lead leg is poised for attack. The cat stance is seen in <u>White Stork Spreads Wings</u>, and many other places in the form.

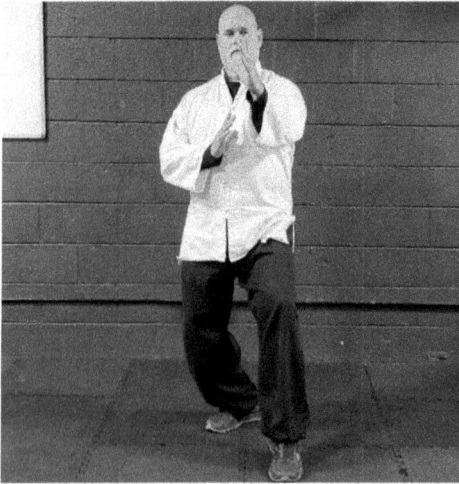

Cat stance (front view) Cat stance (side view)

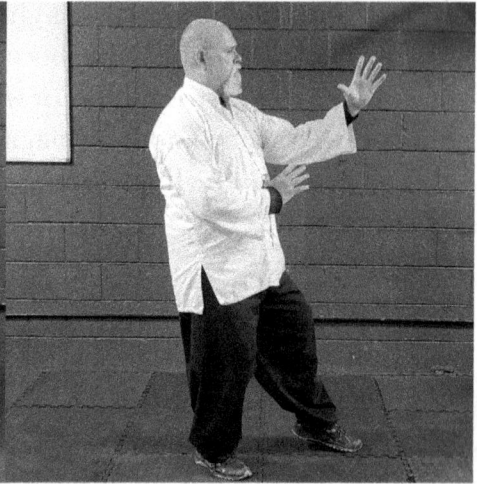

- **Crane stance**. A one-legged stance. The toes of your root leg should be turned out 45 degrees with your knee slightly bent, your hips level. Your other leg is bent at the knee and your knee should be held above the level of your waist. Point the toes down. The raised leg provides some protection to your groin while at the same time facilitating defensive maneuvers and kicks. The hands should be up and protecting your centerline. The crane stance is the least stable stance. The crane stance is seen in maneuvers such as <u>Kick Right</u>.

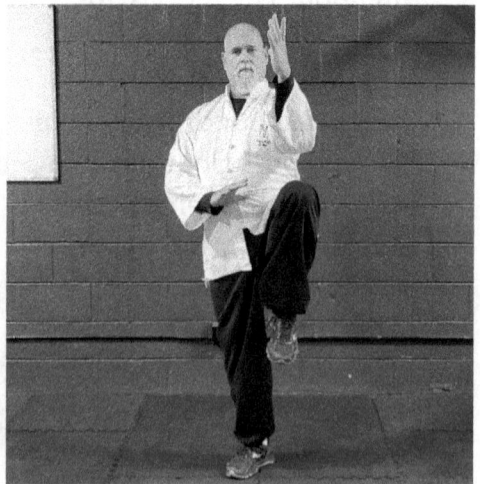

- **Small horse stance**. This is similar to the traditional horse stance but it is less committed; the feet are shoulder width apart and weight is 50/50. This stance is often used in both tai chi and qi gong. It is a less committed stance than the traditional horse stance and easier for new students to practice. The small horse stance is seen in maneuvers such as <u>Commence Tai Chi</u>.

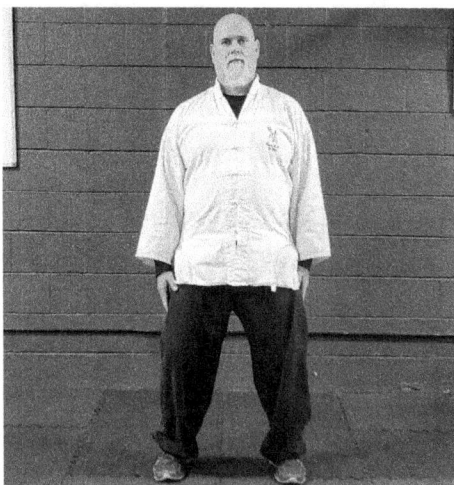

- **60/40 stance** (back, front). 60 percent of your weight should be on your lead leg and both knees are slightly bent. Keep your torso upright, don't bend at the waist. The toes of your lead leg point towards your opponent, the toes of your back leg are turned out 45 degrees. The front knee should not go past the imaginary vertical line of your front toes. To get a feel for how far you can be shifted forward put the toes of your lead foot on a wall and shift your body forward until your knee touches the wall—this is the limit of how far you can go. The 60/40 stance is seen in maneuvers such as <u>Parting the Wild Horses Mane</u>.

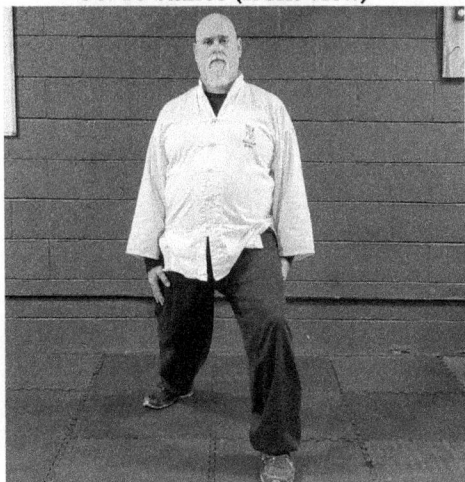

60/40 stance (front view)   **60/40 stance (side view)**

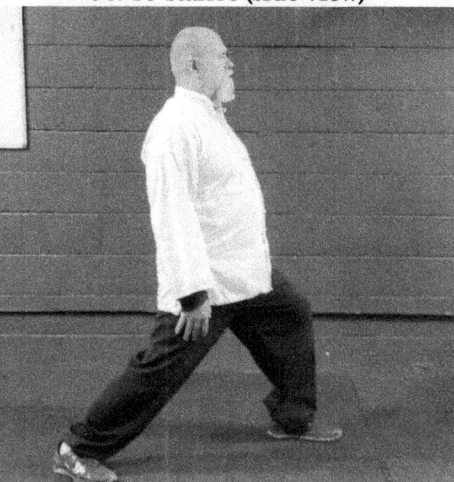

- **Traditional horse stance.** This stance is twice the width of your shoulders, with feet facing forward, weight distribution is 50/50. Knees are bent in the same direction your toes are facing, your hips are level, and your back is straight. This is an excellent stance for strengthening your lower back and legs and for practicing your root. Don't let the top of your head lean behind the imaginary vertical plane created by the back of your heels. The traditional horse stance is not often used in forms, but is an important and frequently used training stance.

Traditional horse stance (front view)   **Traditional horse stance (side view)**

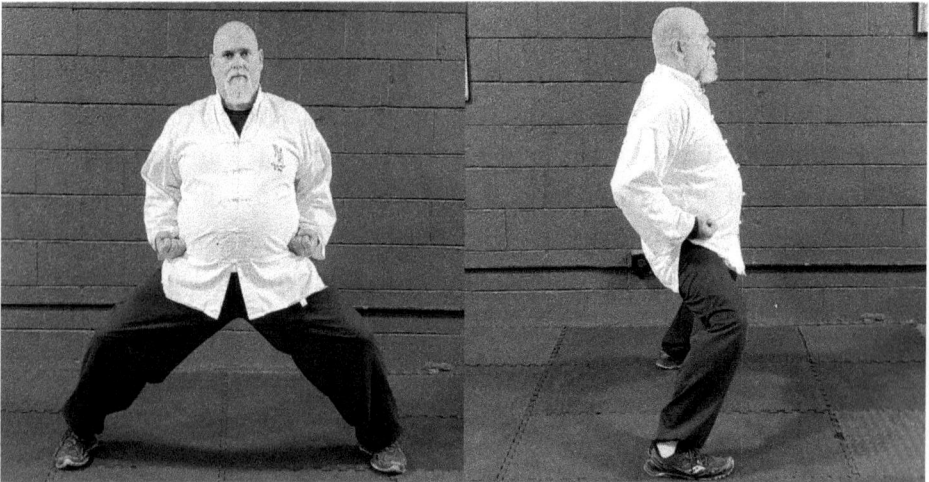

- **Snake creeps low.** Perhaps the most committed stance in tai chi, the weight distribution will depend on how deep your stance is. Your back leg can have anywhere between 60-90 percent of your weight on it. The toes of your back foot are turned out anywhere from 45-90 degrees, and your front foot should be turned in about 30 degrees. Don't bend too far forward at the waist. Although adopting a deep stance will demonstrate an impressive level of flexibility and strength, and may be beneficial to practice, in application a deep snake creeps low stance may be difficult to execute technique from.

Snake creeps low (side view)   Snake creeps low (front view)

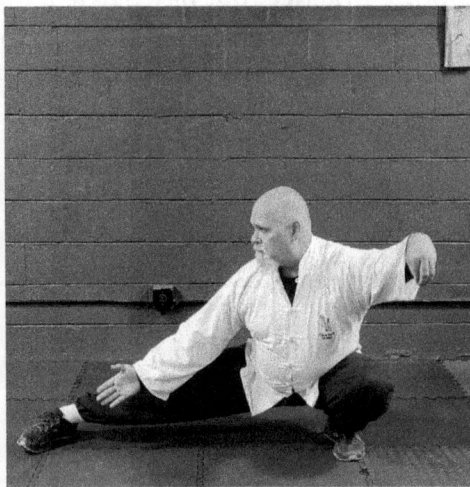

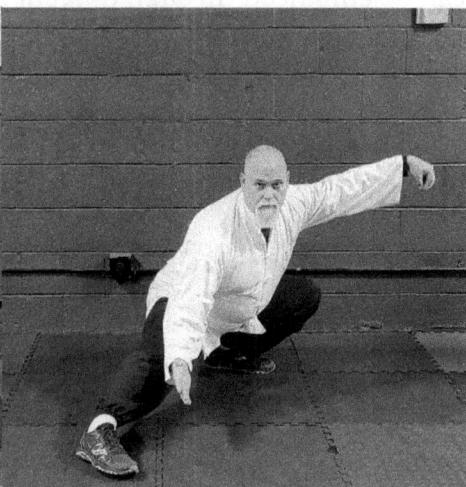

Root

Although there are many skills to practice and develop in tai chi, rooting should be counted as one of the more important ones. Root is defined as the connection between your foot and the ground. It is a relationship that is cultivated by long practice of adopting the correct physical stance, coordinating your breath, setting your intention, and sinking your *qi*. When executing technique, this is where your power and balance originate.

We root through the ball of our feet at the "Bubbling Well" point, KD-1 (description on page 30). Even though we focus on this point practice feeling the ground through your whole foot. Imagine sinking into the ground like the roots of a tree. The further your roots extend, the stronger and more connected you become. Each stance can be enhanced through diligent rooting practice, but pay particular attention to rooting with both the horse stance and the 60/40 stance.

The KD-1 point can also be used to safely expel negative energy into the ground.

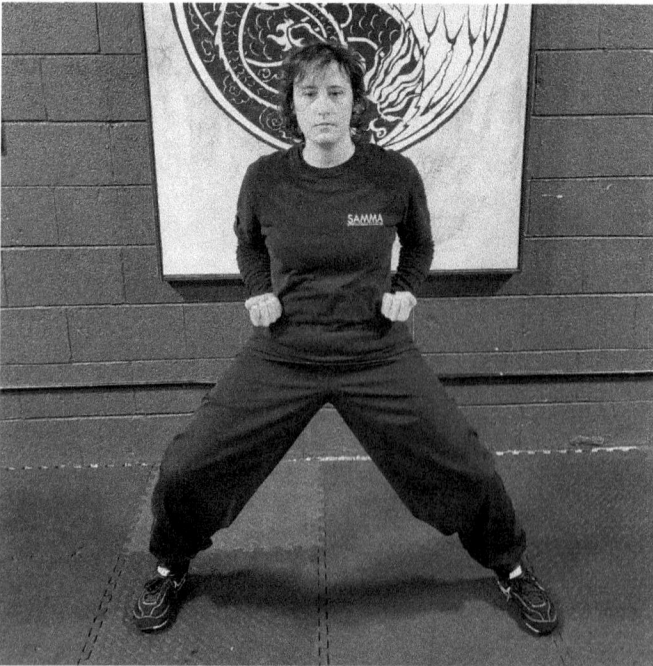

Rooting Practice

The best place to start improving your root is to adopt a horse stance and practice sinking your *qi* through KD-1 into the ground. Start with 30-60 seconds and try to add time each day. Keep your knees bent and your back straight. With each breath imagine your energy sinking and spreading into the ground.

When a partner is available, you can adopt a 60/40 stance with your lead arm held in the wardoff position. Your partner will put both of their hands on your forearm and push toward your back leg. Relax, regulate your breath, and let your structure transmit their force through your body and into the ground through your back foot. If you feel your shoulder start to hurt, stop the exercise and reset. The hurting shoulder indicates that you are pushing back with your muscles which is not the intent of this drill.

Ding

A Chinese word that means something along the lines of "upright" or "erect". It refers to elongating your spine to achieve the best structural alignment. Imagine that you have a rope attached to DU-20 (the top of your head) that is pulling your body upright. To properly manifest ding you need to contrast the upward pull with sinking into KD-1 (the bottom of your feet). If you omit the sinking you risk creating bad structure and allowing yourself to be easily uprooted.

We also use this word while teaching when we want the students to pause at a certain place in the form, usually pausing in a "hold the ball" posture while the instructor makes corrections.

The Three Angles

Although there is some leeway with how you actually place your foot, for the most part, your feet will only ever be at one of three angles relative to the direction of movement—0 degrees, 45 degrees, or 90 degrees. (The one exception to this is when turning in which case you will have to move one of your feet to 135 degrees briefly).

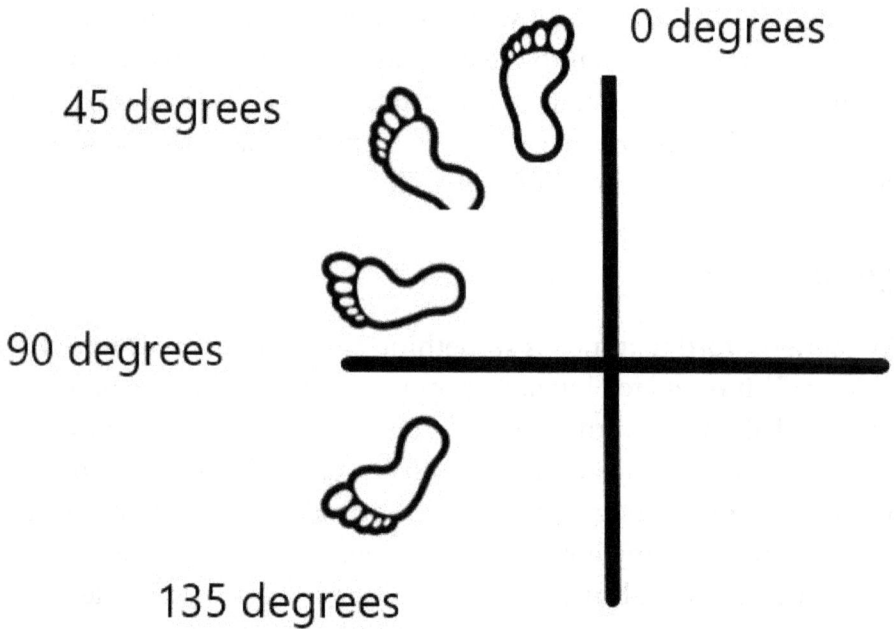

0 degrees

45 degrees

90 degrees

135 degrees

Substantial vs. Insubstantial

Substantial refers to the leg that is weighted, and insubstantial refers to the leg that is unweighted. To stay true to the rules of *yin* and *yang* one has to clearly differentiate between substantial and insubstantial. Additionally, if one does not clearly differentiate this your skill will be low and your techniques will be less effective. Each step you take while practicing should alternate substantial and insubstantial. This is yet another thing to consider when practicing your forms.

Double-Weighted

Being double-weighted refers to a 50/50 weight distribution. This is an undesirable stance. Your weight should constantly be shifting. To hold a double weighted stance will make you slow to react, vulnerable to having your feet swept out from under you, and will stag-

Hand Forms

Dozens of different methods have been developed for hitting with the hands. Some strikes are better suited for hard targets such as bones, and some are better for soft targets like the throat or abdomen. Strikes, grabs, pushes, and pokes are some of the methods done with the fingers and hands. This list is not exhaustive. Included with each is an example from the empty hand forms where the strikes can be found. Proper conditioning should be undertaken prior to hitting anyone with these hand forms or else you risk injury to your fingers, hands, and arms. All things being equal, the smaller the striking surface that is used will transfer greater force into your target.

Hand Forms

2nd MCP. MCP refers to the "metacarpophalangeal joint" and is the anatomical name of the knuckle. This strikes uses the second knuckle as the striking surface. This is most often used to strike your opponent's temples. Seen in <u>Box Tiger at Ears</u>.

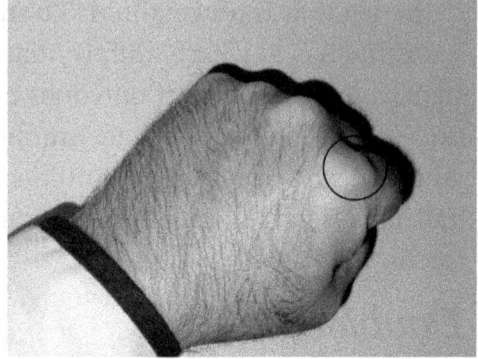

2nd MCP

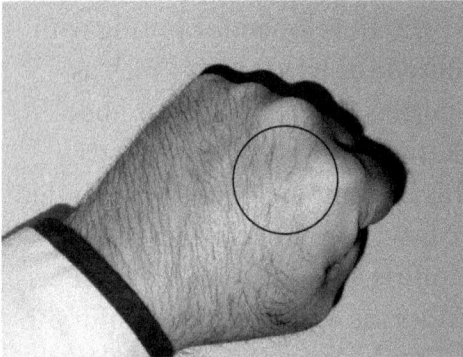

Back fist

Back fist. With the fist held loose, strike with the back of the 2nd and 3rd MCP joints. A common mistake when using this hand form is not turning through your *tan tien* when striking. Seen in <u>Step Up, Deflect, Parry, and Punch</u>.

Buddha palm. A palm strike with the fingers pointing up. The thumb should be extended to the side of the palm, and the palm is slightly cupped. The thumb and index finger should be tense, and the other fingers should be soft. You should also sit the wrist (described on page 111). When striking with the Buddha palm focus on emitting *qi* through PC-8 (described on page 29). Seen in <u>Brush Knee and Twist Step</u>.

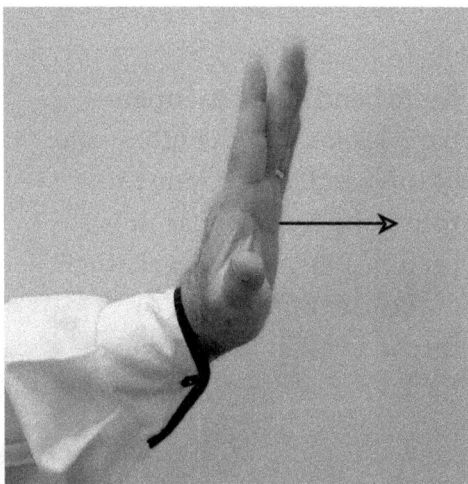

Buddha palm

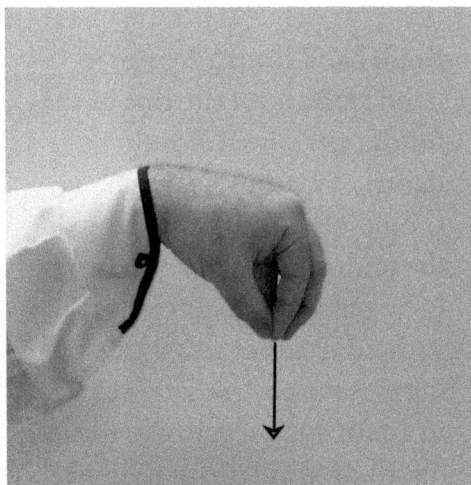

Crane beak

Crane beak. A strike with the tips of all five fingers. The fingers should be held tightly together and should only target soft areas on your opponent's body. It is particularly useful when striking acupressure points. In application your arm is soft like a rope, and your hand is hard. Seen in <u>Single Whip</u>.

Knife hand chop. An open-hand strike with the ulnar side of the hand. The contact surface is the hypothenar. It is used to attack soft targets such as the side of the neck or throat. Seen in Fan Through Back.

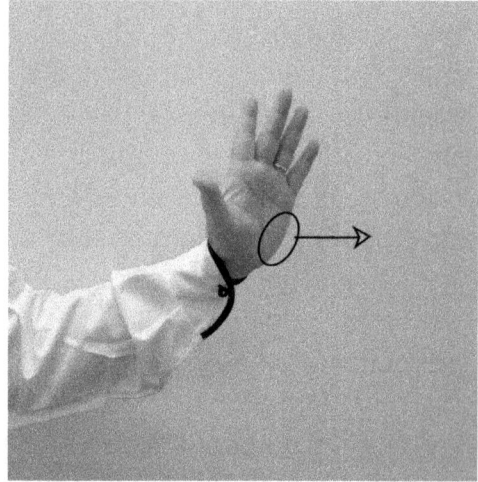

Knifehand chop

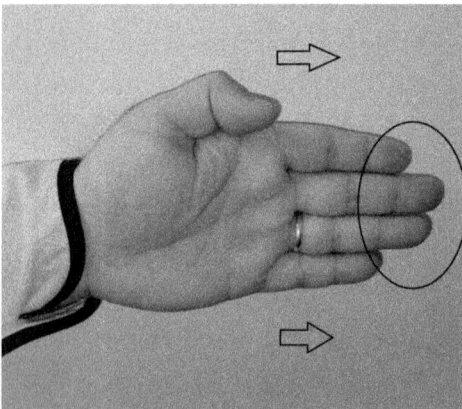

Knifehand thrust

Knife hand thrust. An open hand strike with the tips of the four fingers, held together tightly. The middle finger should be kept slightly bent at the joint so that it is not the only finger that makes contact with your target when executing this strike. Used primarily to attack soft targets like the throat or groin. Seen in Snake Creeps Low.

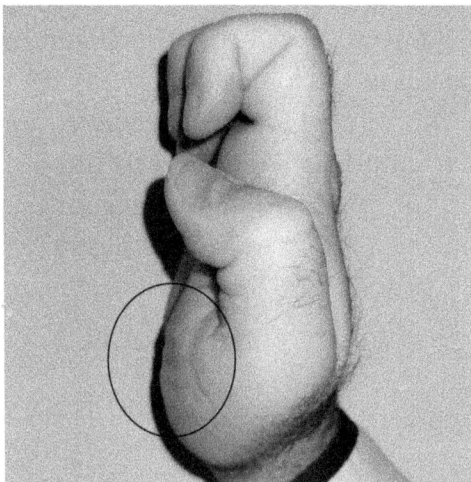

Palm heel. A strike with the base of the open palm. Take care to protect your fingers when striking targets with the palm heel. Often used against the nose, the chin, and the ribs. Seen in <u>High Pat on Horse</u>.

Palm heel

Ridge hand. A strike with the radial side of the palm, usually done with the hand open. The strike should be focused on the space between the thumb and index finger when they are squeezed together. Prior to making contact the wrist should be deviated so as reduce the impact to your wrist joint. Seen in <u>Parting the Wild Horses Mane.</u>

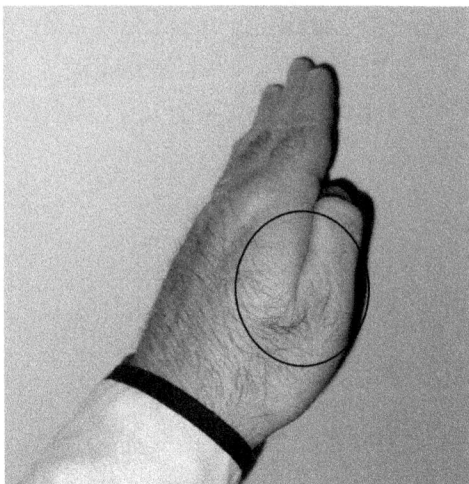

Ridge hand

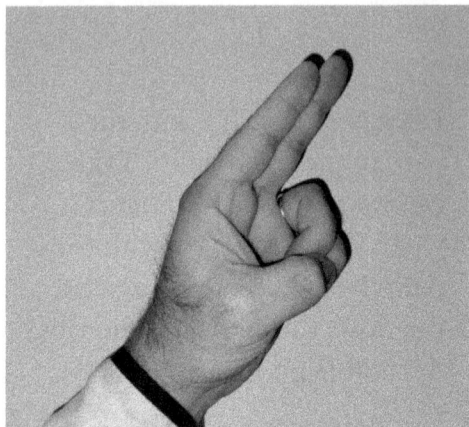

Sword hand. This hand form is seen in the <u>Tai Chi Sword</u> forms. Your thumb touches the fingernails of the first two fingers. The sword hand form is used as a counterbalance to the fact that your other hand is holding a sword. It is also used for aesthetic reasons.

Sword hand

Tai chi fist. A loose fist (as opposed to a tightly held fist as seen in kung fu). The bones in the hand should be in line with the radius and ulna bones in the forearm. The striking surface is the front of the 2nd and 3rd MCP joints. Seen in <u>Apparent Withdrawal</u>.

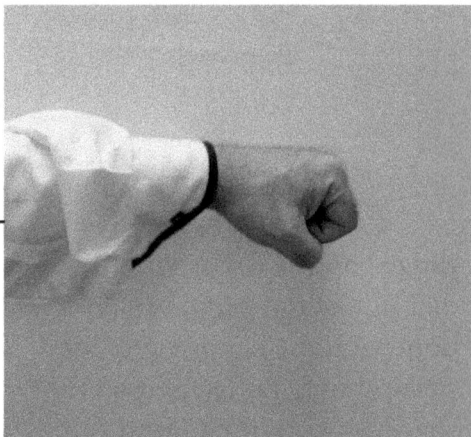

Tai chi fist

Kicks

Kicking in tai chi can look different than kicking in most other martial arts. The intention is often that your opponent impale themselves on your outstretched foot instead of using your force to strike them with your foot, taking advantage of their momentum.

Kicks generally go through four stages. The first is the chamber, the second is the execution of the kick, the third is the re-chamber, and the final stage brings the kicking leg back into the original starting position.

Kicks can be practiced in the air (without a partner), with a partner holding a kicking shield, or with a hanging or floor mounted heavy bag.

- **Crescent kick.** This kick moves in a circle (from the hip joint). The side of the foot is the striking surface. This is the most difficult kick to perform in tai chi.

- **Heel kick.** A type of front kick that uses the heel as the striking surface. Mostly targeting the head or face.

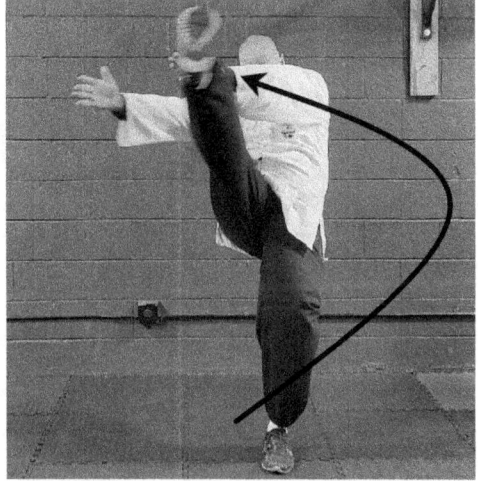

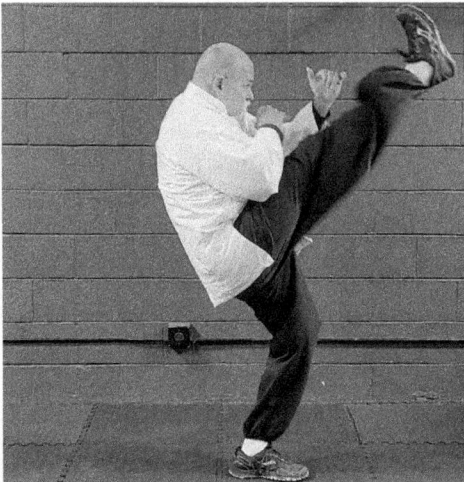

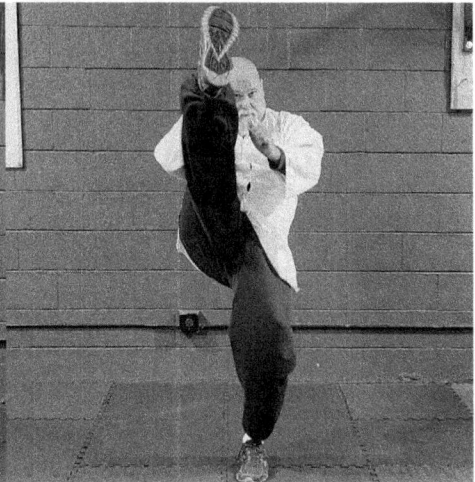

- **Toe kick** A type of front kick that uses the toes as the striking surface. Keep your toes, foot, knee, leg, and hips lined up directly with your target. Alternately, the top of the foot or the ball of the foot can also be used.

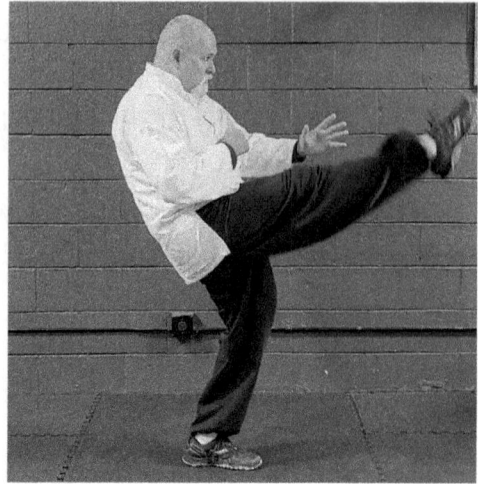

Holding a Ball

A multipurpose posture that is used as a transition, a preparatory or chambering move, and an exercise. The posture adopts a cat stance with the hands held as if you are holding an imaginary beach ball on one side of your body. If the ball is to be held on the right side, the left leg will be forward and the left hand will be palm up at your right hip. The right hand will be palm down at the right shoulder. Your head and left foot will be oriented toward your imaginary opponent, and your right foot, hips, and shoulders will be 45 degrees offline turned to the right. Keep your shoulders relaxed and your elbows down.

As a group instructional aid, we use this as a stopping point when learning the forms. Many of the movements will transition through the "hold a ball" posture. As a result, it makes a natural stopping point.

For applications, the hand that is by your hip is chambered, allowing maximum space for acceleration for executing hand techniques. This posture is often adopted as a prelude to wardoff.

As an exercise, we practice shifting the ball from right to left from both a static posture and while practicing tai chi walking.

Note the alignment of the weight-bearing leg (the root leg) and the toes. It is important to keep this knee and toe alignment any time you are putting weight on one of your legs to get proper structure as well as to prevent injury.

Your hips are aligned to the same direction as your root leg. The foot of your lead leg is pointing in the direction of movement. Your head and eyes are directed towards the front.

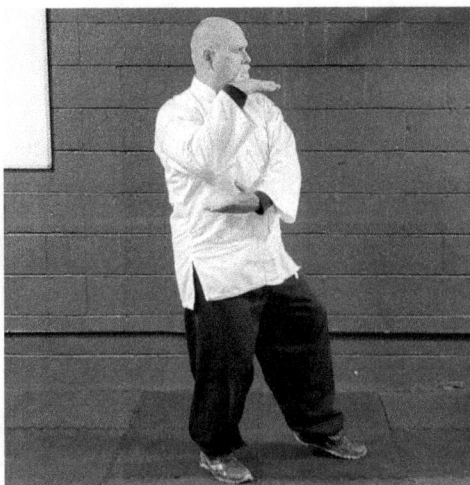

Hold Right Ball (side view)   Hold Right Ball (front view)

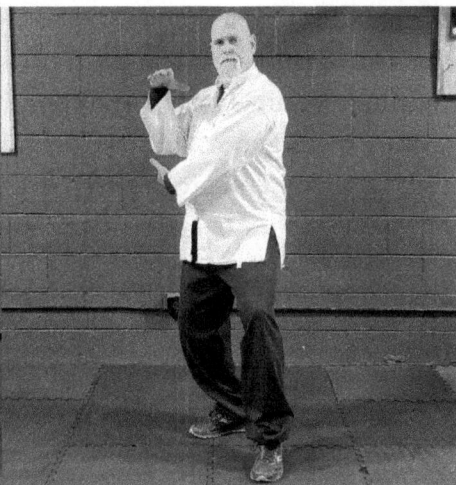

Opening and Closing the Kua

The *kua* is essentially the inguinal crease, although it can refer to the function of the hip joint as well. The *kua* can be either opened or closed and is dictated by what you are trying to accomplish. The *kua* helps us to create structure in our body and is an important part of the power generation chain that starts with the feet. Kicks, movement, and stances are intimately connected with the *kua*. For example, to perform a front kick the *kua* of the root leg must be opened. When adopting a crane stance, the kua of the root leg is open and the *kua* of the leg that is held up is closed. When we perform tai chi walking, we alternately are opening and closing the *kua* on both sides. Power generation requires force, originating from the connection between your foot and the ground, extending through your *kua*, guided up to your *tan tien*, and out your arm.

The pictures below show the closing of the *kua* from a 60/40 stance as seen from the front. **1**. Keeping the left foot fully on the floor, rotate it 45 degrees to the right, letting the knee move to the right at the same time. **2**. This picture shows the stance with the *kua* closed.

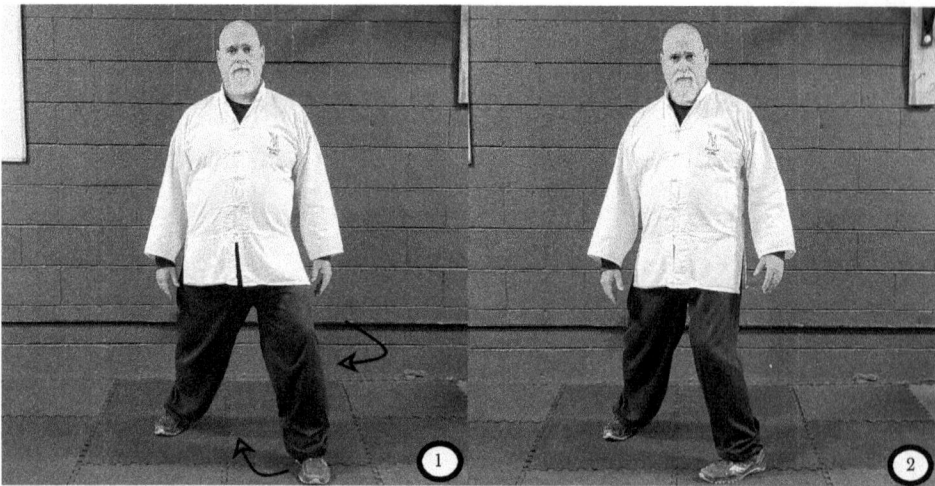

Closing the kua

The pictures below show the closing of the *kua* from a 60/40 stance as viewed from the side. **1**. Shows a 60/40 stance with the *kua* open. **2**. Shows the *kua* closed.

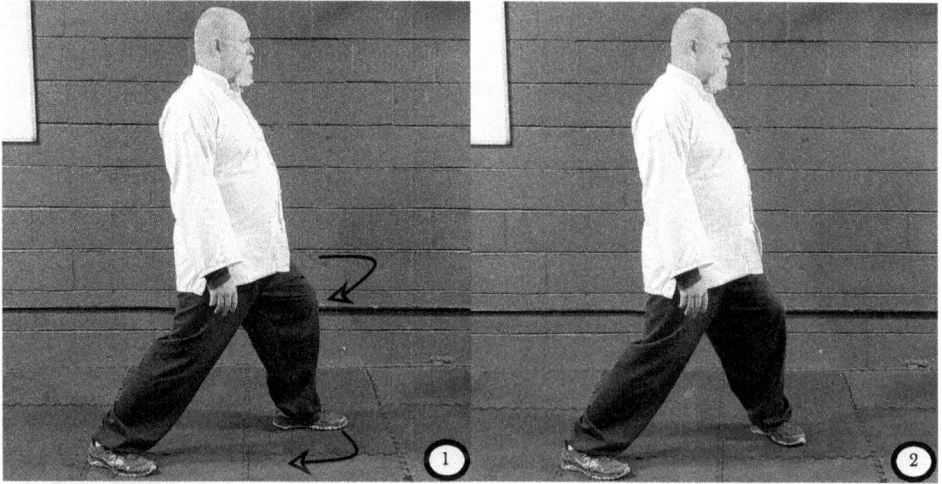

The pictures below show opening the *kua* while walking forward. **1**. From a 60/40 stance with your weight over the left foot, rock back and shift your weight over your right foot allowing the toes of the left foot to raise. Open your left hip to the left allowing the left foot and knee to follow. **2**. Shift your weight forward onto the left foot. Keep your right heel on the ground.

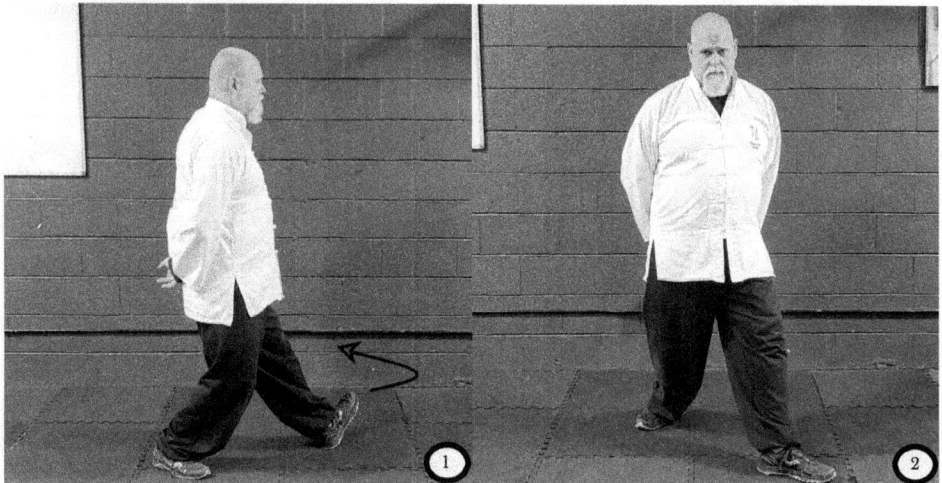

Movement

Movement in tai chi is quite technical and nuanced; it was designed to facilitate the application of proper technique while maneuvering, reacting, kicking, and applying techniques during hand-to-hand combat.

Tai chi step. The basic method of locomotion in tai chi. **1**. Start with feet together. **2**. Take a natural step forward, lead with the heel of the left foot. **3**.Rock forward, shifting your weight onto the whole foot. Keep both heels down and sinking into the ground. Knees stay soft and slightly bent. Shift your weight forward onto your left foot until 60 percent of your weight has shifted onto it. **4**. Next shift your weight onto your right leg, allowing the toes of your left foot to lift. Don't let your knee extend beyond the vertical plane created by your toes.

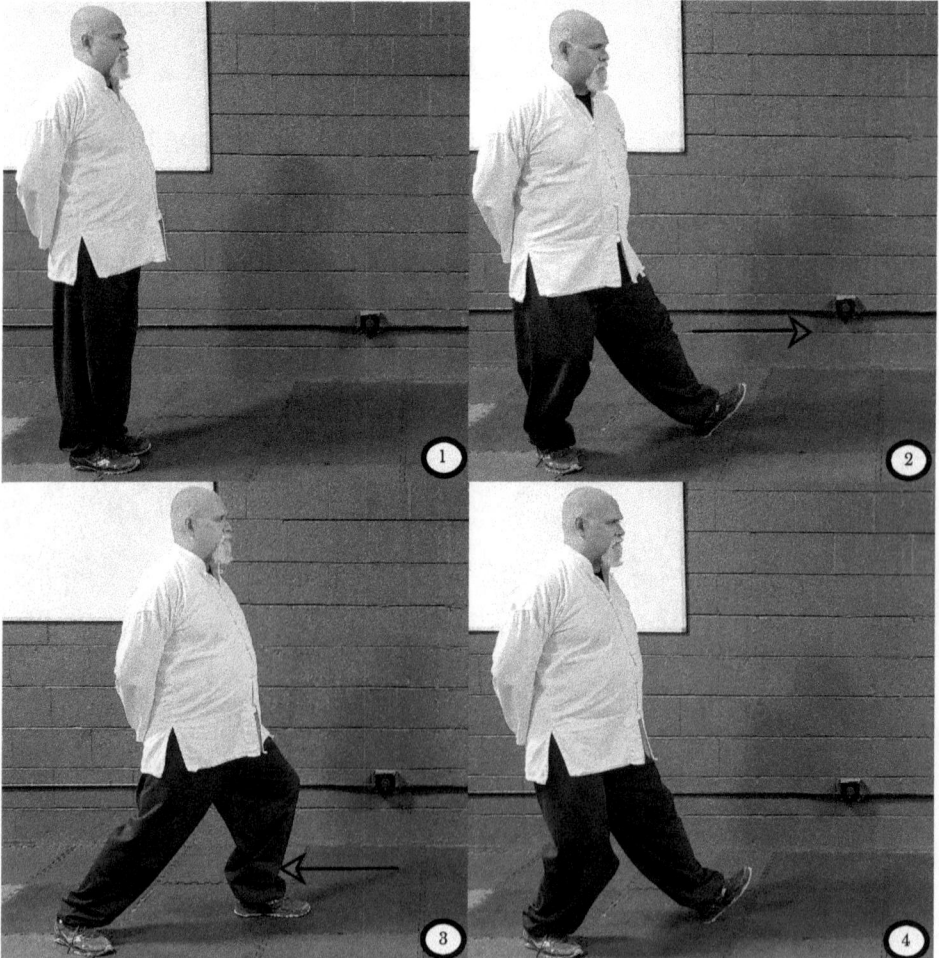

5. Open your left *kua* by rotating your hips to the left, this will simultaneously close your right *kua*. Some students think of this in terms of moving the left foot or rotating from the heel, but this is not correct. This movement should originate in the *kua*. Your left toes should now be facing 30-45 degrees to the left of the direction you are moving.

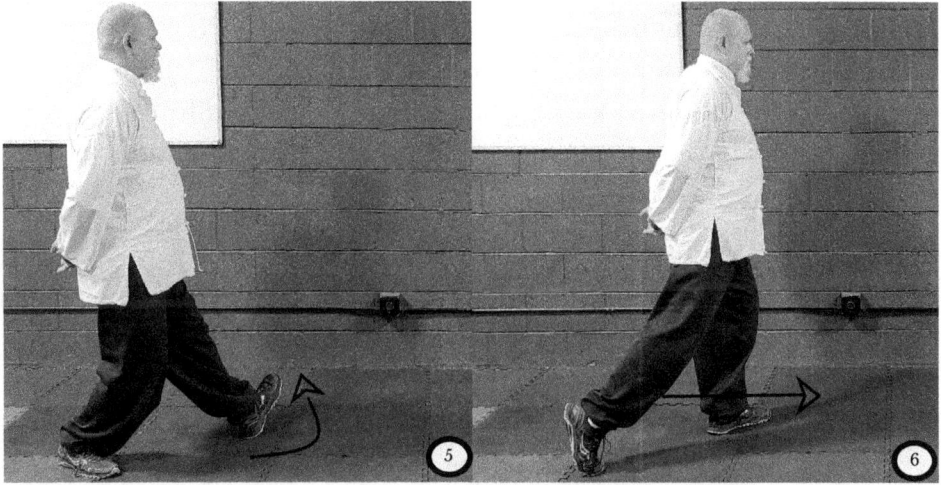

6. Next, push off your right foot allowing your weight to shift onto the left foot. Your right heel will come up. **7.** The final part is to lift your right foot and take a step forward to begin the process once again on the other side. This last step should be done with your hips in a generally neutral and forward-facing position. Don't let your knees come together as you take your step. With each step practice sinking your *qi* into the ground through both feet. The goal is to feel relaxed and balanced throughout the entire movement.

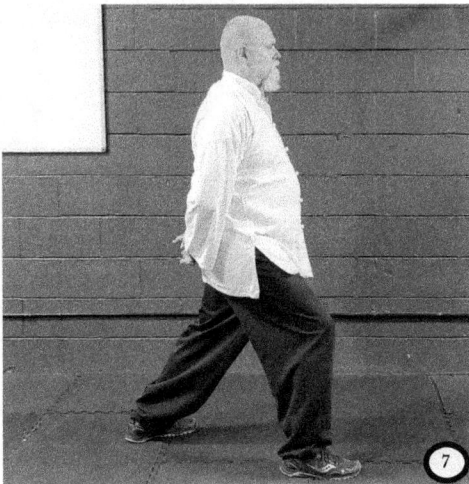

The following steps are variations of the above-described tai chi step.

Half step. This step moves your body forward only half the distance of your normal stride. It ends with a retrograde motion that has its own defensive properties. **1.** From attention, start by shifting your weight to your right leg. This allows you to lift your right heel without losing your balance. **2.** Take a natural step with your left leg leading with your left heel, toes up. **3.** Shift your weight onto your left foot and settle into a 60/40 stance. **4.** Continue shifting your weight forward onto your left leg. Let your right heel lift up.

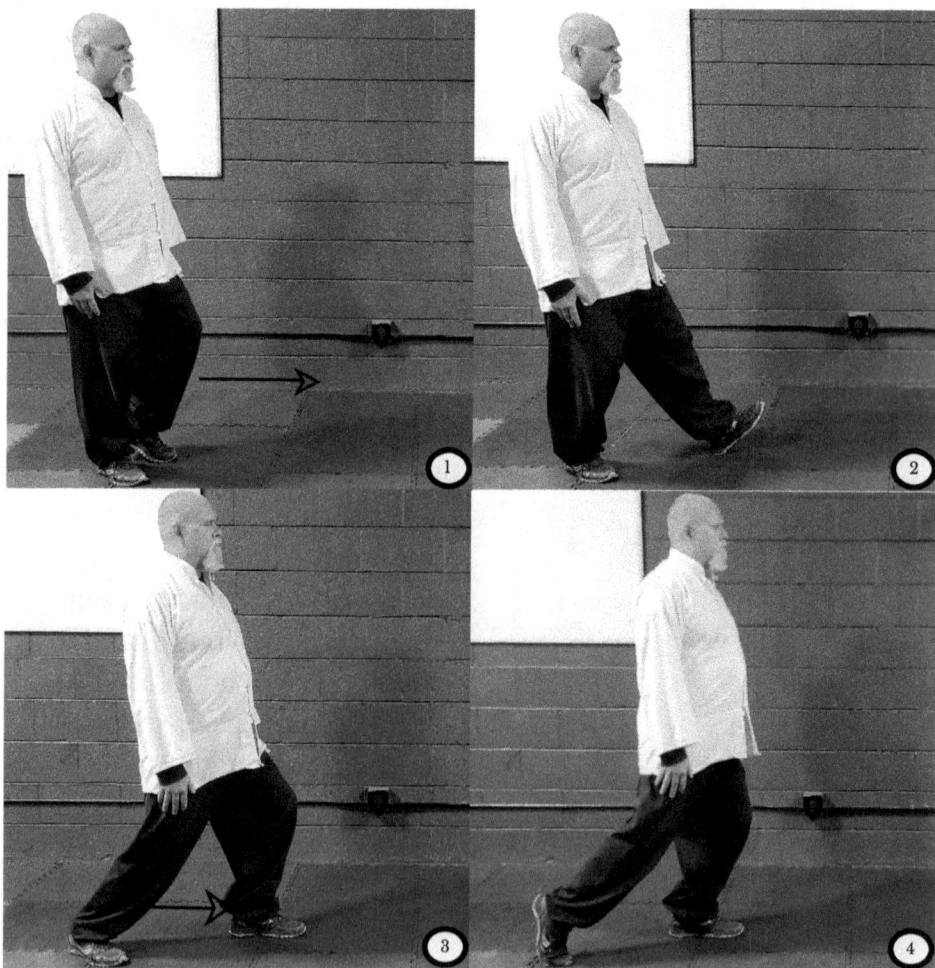

5. Bring the toes of your right foot approximately to the level of your left heel. 6. Settle back onto your right foot and move into a left leg forward cat stance. 7. Pick up your left foot and take a step, leading with your heel. 8. Shift your weight onto the left foot ending in a 60/40 stance. Seen in the transition between <u>Parting the Wild Horses Mane</u> and <u>White Stork Spreads Wings</u>.

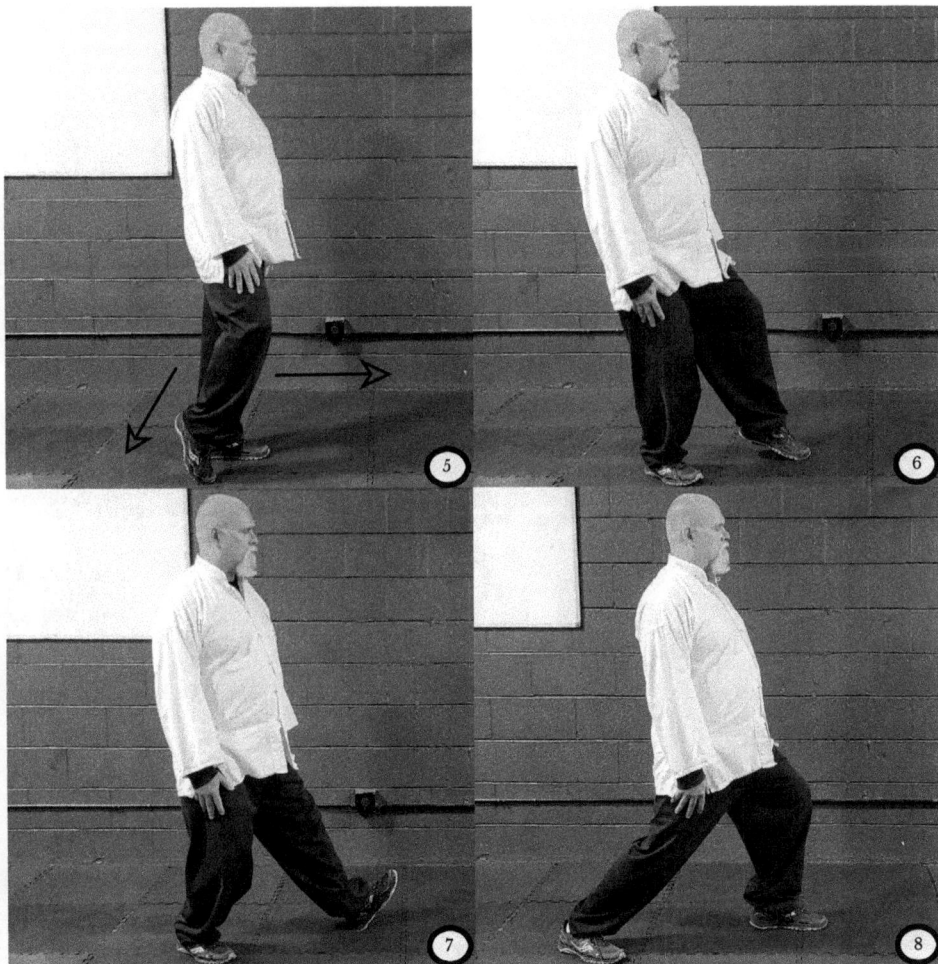

Back step. A method of moving backwards away from your opponent. **1.** Start with your feet together. Lift your left leg bringing the knee above the level of your waist. **2.** Step backwards with the left foot and bring the left toes onto the ground. It may take some practice to take this step and feel balanced. Keep your right knee slightly bent and sink your *qi* into the ground to firmly establish your root. **3.** Shift your weight onto the left foot, briefly establishing a 60/40 stance. **4.** Shift your weight onto your left foot, lift your right heel.

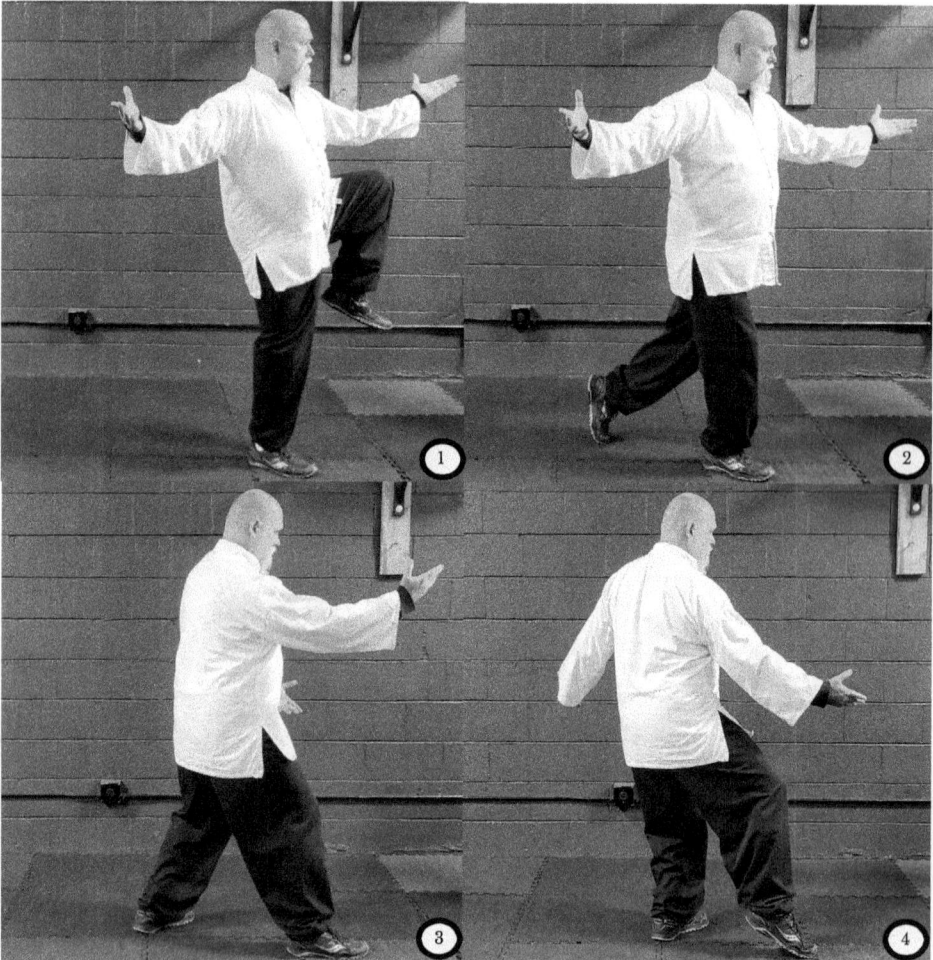

5. Lift your right leg bringing your knee above the level of your waist. **6**. Take a step backwards with your right foot. **7**. Shift your weight backwards onto your right foot ending in a 60/40 stance. Seen in <u>Step Back and Repulse Monkey</u>.

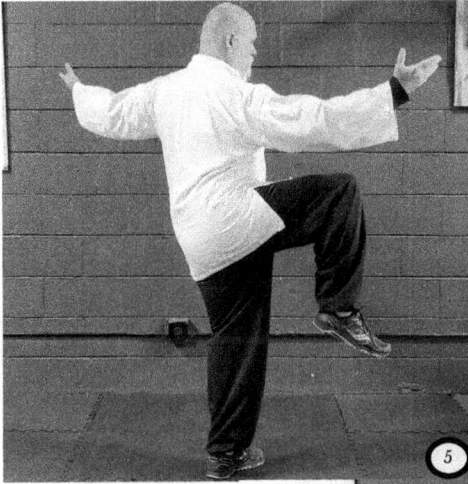

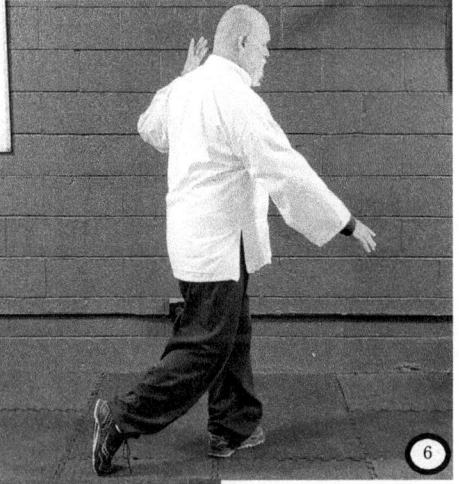

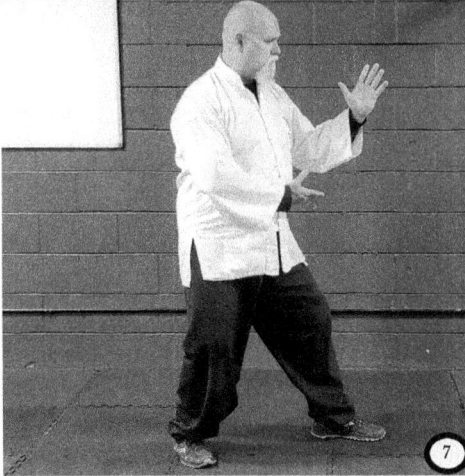

Side Step. A method of moving from side-to-side. **1.** Start with your feet together. **2.** Shift your weight to your right foot. This allows you to lift your left heel without falling over. **3.** Step to the left approximately one shoulder width distance. Place your left toes on the ground. **4.** Shift your weight onto your left leg, bringing the left heel down.

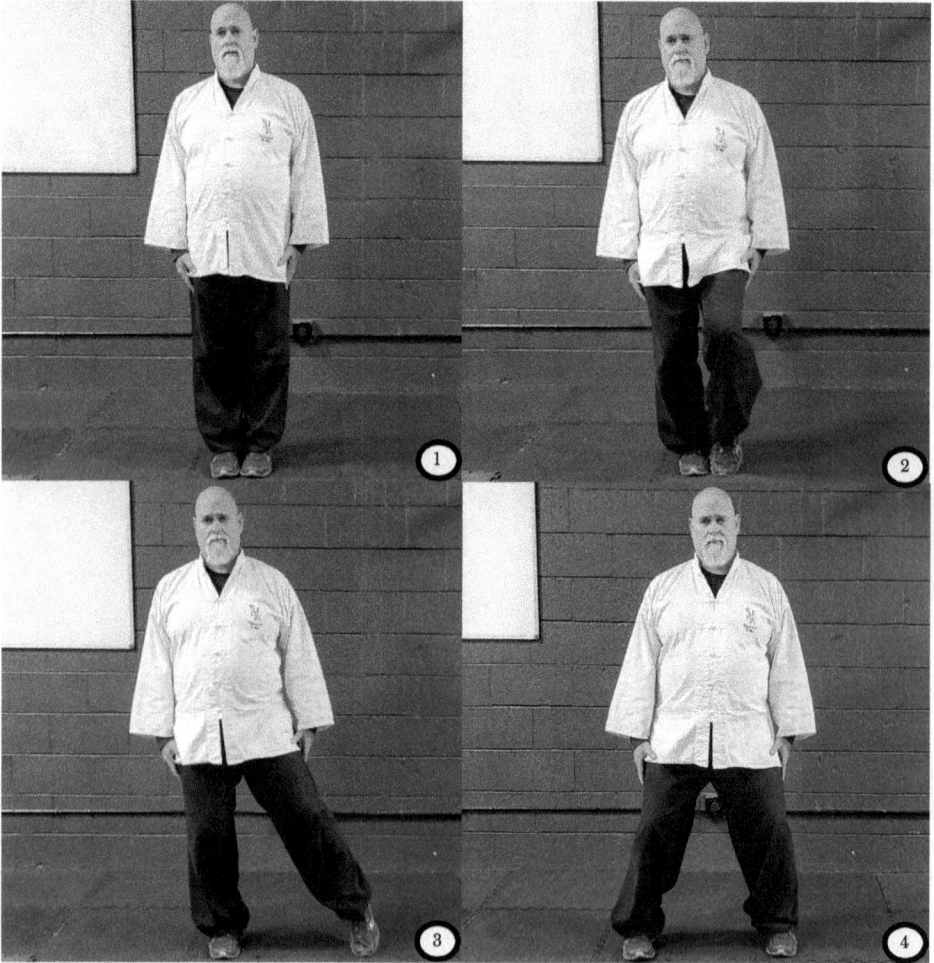

5. Continue shifting your weight onto your left foot. Once your weight is on the left foot lift up your right heel. **6.** Complete the step to the left by bringing your right foot next to your left. Place your right foot down next to your left foot, toes first. Lastly drop your right heel. Seen in maneuvers such as <u>Wave Hands Like Clouds</u>.

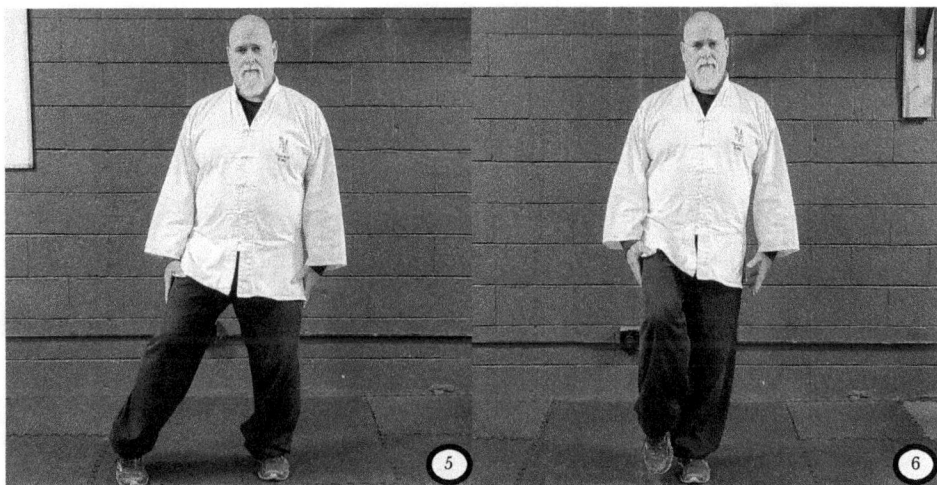

Turning 180 degrees. A method of turning 180 degrees. **1.** Begin the turn at the end of the forward motion of your step, you are in a left foot forward 60/40 stance. **2.** Shift your weight to your right foot and lift the toes of your left foot.

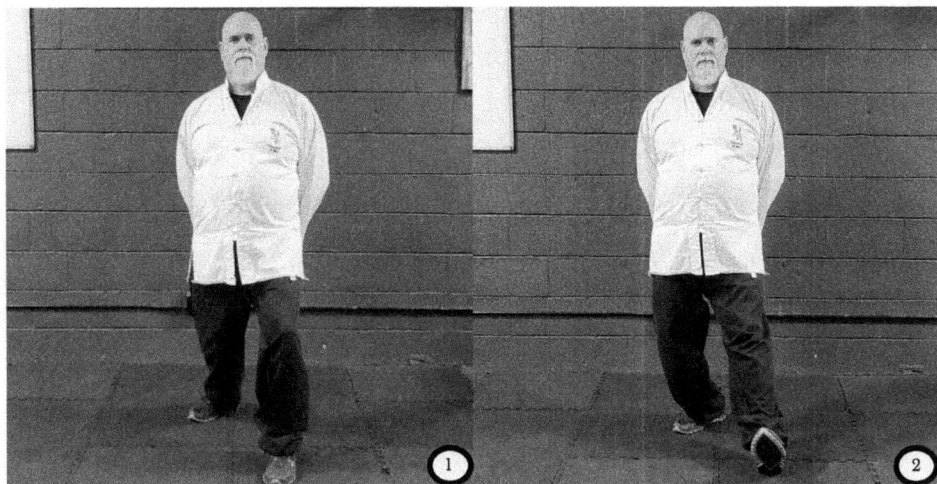

3. Turn your left foot inward on the heel approximately 135 degrees and put the toes down. Turn your hips to the right. You should feel a line of tension on the outside of your right leg. **4**. Shift your weight to the left leg. You will now feel a line of tension in your left leg.

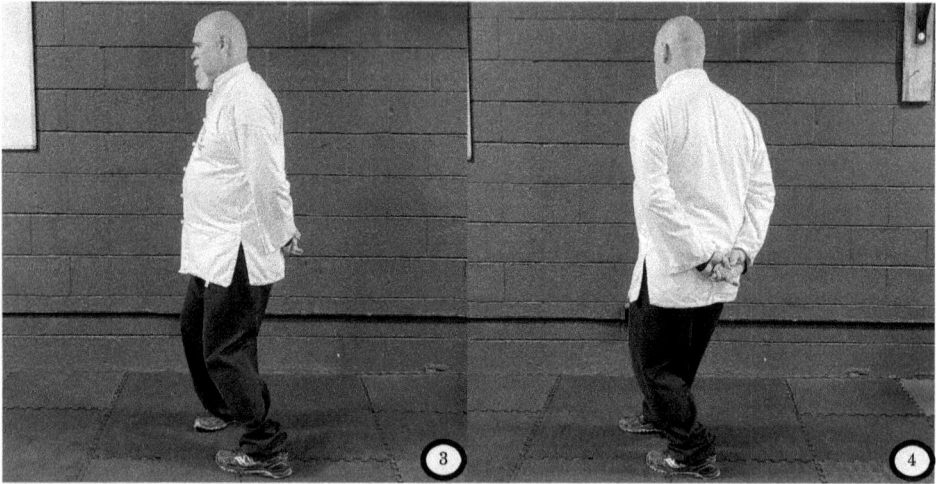

5. Lift your right heel and unwind this tension by turning on the ball of your right foot. Continue to turn your hips until they face in the new direction of travel, **6**. Lift your right foot up (it is now your lead) and take a step in the new direction of movement. Seen in the transition between <u>Fan Through Back</u> and <u>Step Up, Deflect, Parry and Punch</u>.

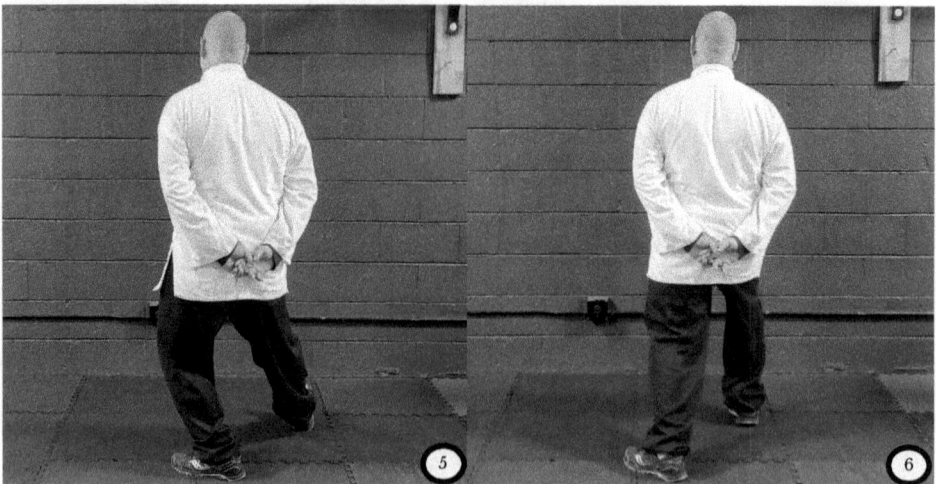

Momentum

Momentum is a scientific unit of measurement that is of particular consequence to the study of tai chi. It is the product of an object's mass multiplied by its velocity. When we move, we are generating momentum. When consciously directed, momentum allows the tai chi practitioner to transmit force efficiently; when it is not consciously directed our tai chi becomes unfocused and limited.

One way of directing momentum is to bring awareness to all of the movements our body is making. Feeling our feet connecting to the ground through KD-1. Sinking into our postures as we transition from one stance to the next. Flexing and extending our knees to capitalize on the potential energy created through this process, to guide the momentum through our *tan tien*, into and up our spine, through the shoulder, elbow, and wrist joint, and finally out through the hand.

As your hands perform the various strikes and deflections pay close attention to the pathing. You want to avoid moving your hands in a way that forces you to either stop or reverse their direction of travel. Additionally, you want to limit the amount of muscle tension needed to execute techniques. Rely instead on momentum starting from your root (primarily the back foot) directed by your *tan tien*. Your arms are simply the conduit for the transmission of force.

We study and practice the forms to access the proper principles of movement, rooting, breath, and structure contained within.

Extending the knee joint by pressing into the ground sends the energy to our *tan tien* where it is directed to the appropriate target via hands, elbows, shoulders, or feet. Spurious or unconscious movement has momentum, but it is undesirable and inefficient. Undirected movements are not good tai chi.

Muscle tension can inhibit the flow of *qi*, limit the transfer of power, and can lead to structural misalignment. All of these detriments can in turn negatively influence momentum. It is one of the reasons we are forever trying to learn how to relax. When practicing any of the forms, exercises, or drills you should be seeking areas of tension in your body and finding ways to get them to relax. Breathe and relax.

Wave Hands Momentum Drill. From the <u>Wave Hands Like Clouds</u> posture, establish your root and practice moving your hands through interlocking circles in front of your body. Do the following circular hand motions slowly—concentrate on turning your waist side to side to move your hands left and right without using any arm muscles. Then, focus to how your hands can move through the downward side of the circles using only the effect of gravity. Next, on the upward arc of the circles, pay attention to which of the muscles in your arm are required to lift your hands. After a few repetitions, move your waist to the side quickly and forcibly to get your hands to complete the interlocking circles with momentum. This can be done statically or dynamically. When practicing this while stepping to the side, practice leading force from your foot, into your *tan tien,* and out through your arms. There are many variations to this drill.

Sitting the Wrist

Although we strive for relaxation and ease of movement in tai chi, one small exception to this is what we refer to as "sitting the wrist". There are some postures that require our wrist to be extended so that a line of tension is created along the back of the wrist joint. This is sometimes done when the palm faces out with the fingers pointing up as when performing a palm strike, and sometimes it is done with the palm facing down and the fingers facing forward as seen at the end of Commence Tai Chi.

Tai Chi Walking

Tai chi walking is primarily used as a warm-up or training event. Tai chi walking gives students an opportunity to practice specific skills in isolation such as integrating proper breathing with their movements or improving the coordination of hands and feet. Many drills can be done while practicing tai chi walking to include elements from silk reeling, specific postures from the empty hand forms, transitions between techniques, and even practicing elements from the weapons forms.

Skills to focus on while practicing tai chi walking include—sinking qi through both feet as you move into each stance, proper breath, identifying areas where you are holding stress and tension and relaxing them, hand and foot coordination, generating and circulating *qi*, opening and closing the *kua*, keeping your head up and your eyes engaged, breath and body integration, balance, smooth transitions, movement without stopping, and many others.

Points of Attention During Practice

The following describes specific areas to pay attention to while practicing tai chi and is equally applicable to warm-ups, drills, and the forms.

- **Hands and wrists**. Primarily refers to your palm and fist. With the palm strike, your thumb is pushed out and your middle finger sets in slightly. Palm is cupped and you should sit the wrist. Your fist is held like you have a ping-pong ball inside. The fist has to stay relaxed for *qi* to circulate. An open palm is *yang*, a closed fist is *yin*. We say, "Sit the wrist and extend the fingers". Although the open palm and the closed fist are the most common hand forms, there are others. Each has its own qualities and characteristics.

- **Elbows and shoulders**. Sink the shoulders and drop your elbows. Keep the muscles loose and relaxed. Tension takes away power and causes stagnation. Keeping the elbows down also prevents someone from striking your HT-1, a *dim mak*, or acupuncture point. The tops of the trapezius muscles are a common place where stress and tension are held.

- **Head**. The head is held upright. Eyes gaze at nothing in particular but slightly precede the movements of the action (or *yang*) hand. Your head is held like it's suspended from a rope that extends to the sky. Relax the tension in your neck.

- **Chest**. Don't pluck out your chest. Keep it soft and rounded. Relax your abdomen and breathe from your *tan tien*.

- **Waist, hips, and thighs**. Your waist is the steering wheel that redirects your enemy's attacks. The tops of your pelvis should be level with the ground. Don't bend at the waist while executing techniques. When you move into a stance clearly differentiate where your weight is. Avoid becoming double-weighted, with your weight distribution 50/50.

- **Legs, knees, and feet**. Don't tense the muscles, but your legs can't be like noodles. My teacher says, "Relaxed but not quite relaxed". The knee should not go past the toe. Legs should never completely straighten. You should almost never have a 50/50 weight distribution. Feet are the root of all postures. Keep *yi* focused on the bottom of foot, or root. *Qi* must be able to reach KD-1. When loading weight onto your leg it is important to keep the toes and the kneecap pointed in the same direction, otherwise you risk injury to your knee joint. Some turns are done on the heel, and some are done on the ball of the foot. This small point will have significant impact on your movement and technique if done incorrectly.

- **Be soft**. Let go of tension. Relax tight muscles.

- **Go slow**. Don't move too fast. Moving too fast hides mistakes and poor technique.

- **Continuous motion**. Once you begin the form, your whole body should be in motion without identifiable breaks.

- **Clearly differentiate between Yin and Yang**. Tai chi is the physical embodiment of *Yin/Yang* Theory. All of our moves should comply with these rules.

- **Breathe**. Forward or downward motion, exhale. Backward or upward motion inhale.

- **Clear your mind and focus on the circulation of qi**. Feel *qi* accumulating in your *tan tien*.

- **Be smooth**. Avoid jagged or disjointed movements.

Points of Attention During Practice

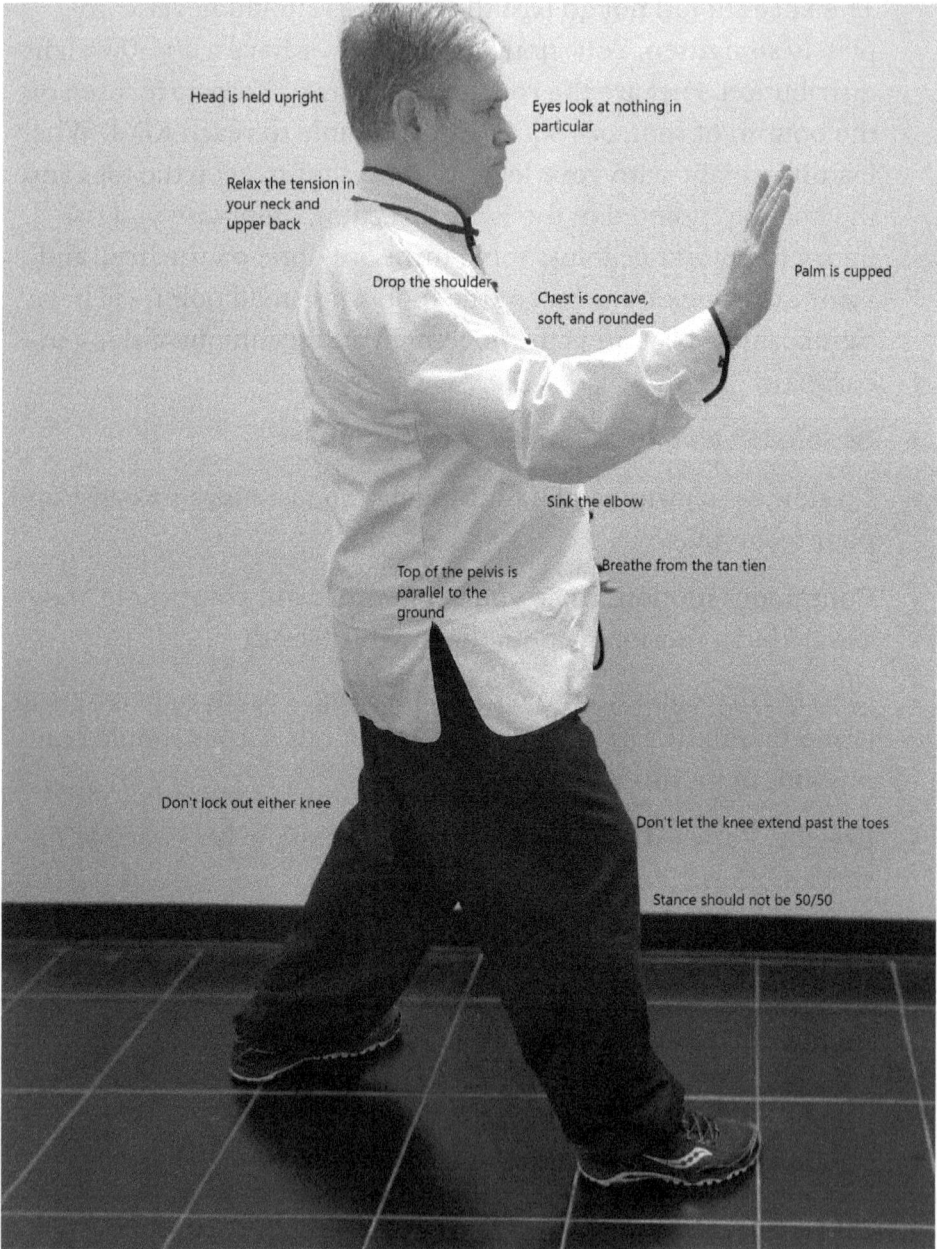

Head is held upright

Eyes look at nothing in particular

Relax the tension in your neck and upper back

Drop the shoulder

Chest is concave, soft, and rounded

Palm is cupped

Sink the elbow

Top of the pelvis is parallel to the ground

Breathe from the tan tien

Don't lock out either knee

Don't let the knee extend past the toes

Stance should not be 50/50

Training
and Development

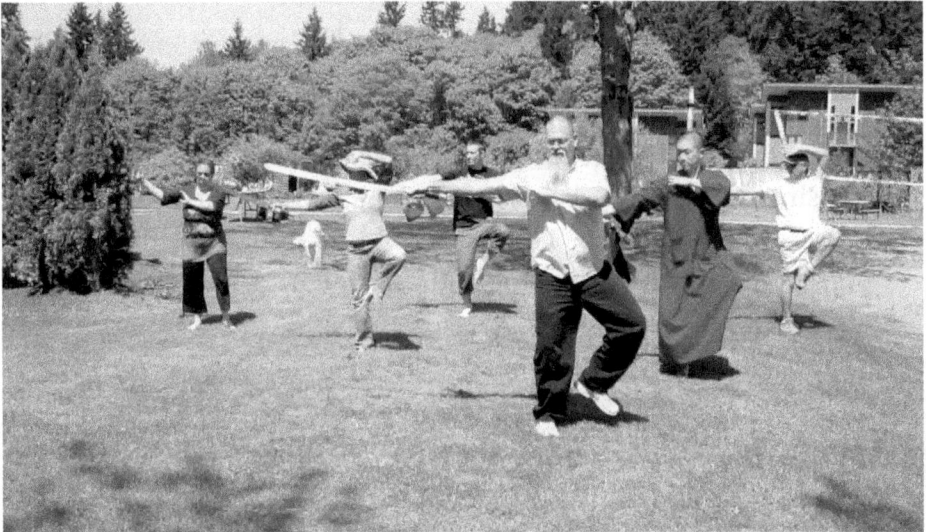

Tai Chi Saber Class

Bastyr University

2013

Drills

There are many types of drills in tai chi; There are solo, partner, and bag drills, static and dynamic drills, and drills to develop *jing* and sensitivity. A complete description of all the drills that are used is beyond the scope of this book. Some of the more helpful ones are described below.

Physical Skills

- **Elevator hands.** Partner Drill. **1.** <u>Student One</u> starts with their hands in front of their stomach, palms down, fingers extending forward. <u>Student Two</u> places their palms on the backs of <u>Student One's</u> hands. **2.** <u>Student One</u> will then move their hands randomly but slowly and <u>Student Two</u> has to stay in contact. Increasing the speed and altering the trajectory of the movements increases the difficulty. This drill provides students with the opportunity to practice sticking and listening *jing*.

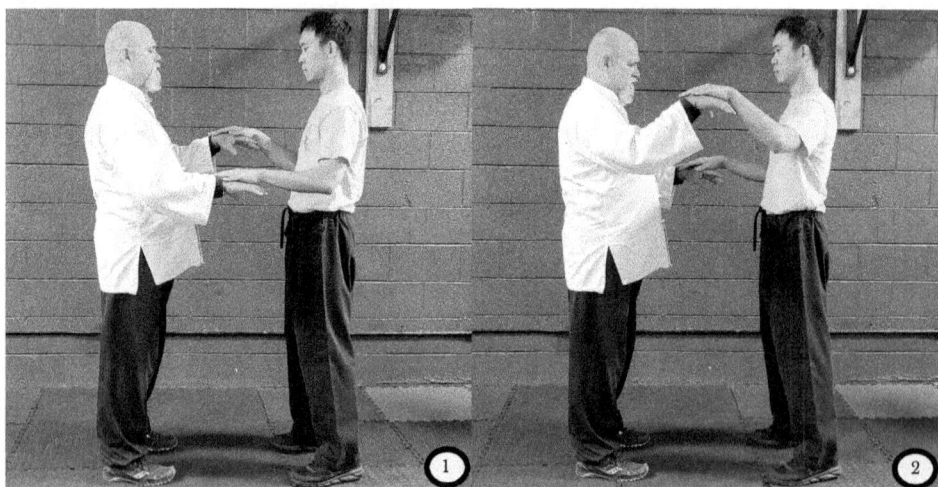

- **Shooting palm.** **1.** Start in a traditional horse stance. Keep your feet stationary. Move your right upturned palm forward, crossing your centerline towards your left shoulder. **2.** Turn your hips to the left. Your right hand moves forward and up to the level of your shoulder. Your left hand remains chambered at your left hip.

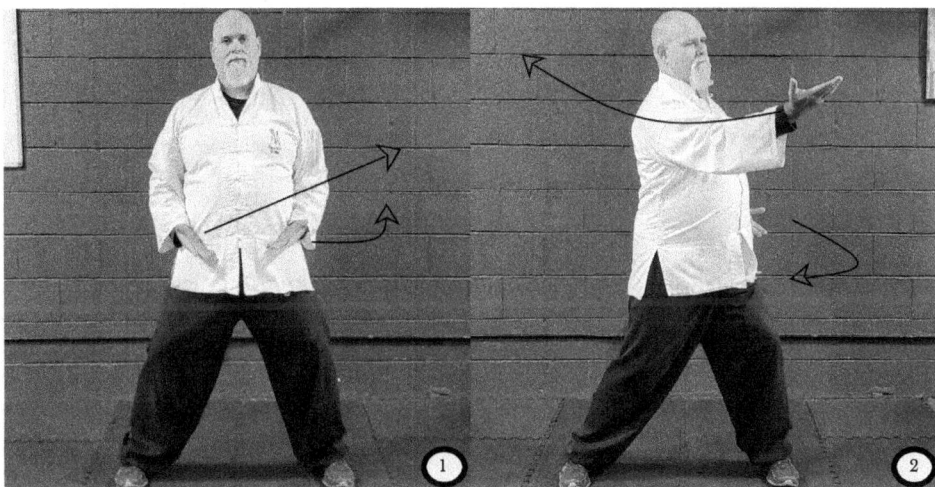

3. Turn your hips to the right, bringing your right arm up and back. **4.** The right hand spirals up until your hand is over your head palm facing up. Your hips turn to the left.

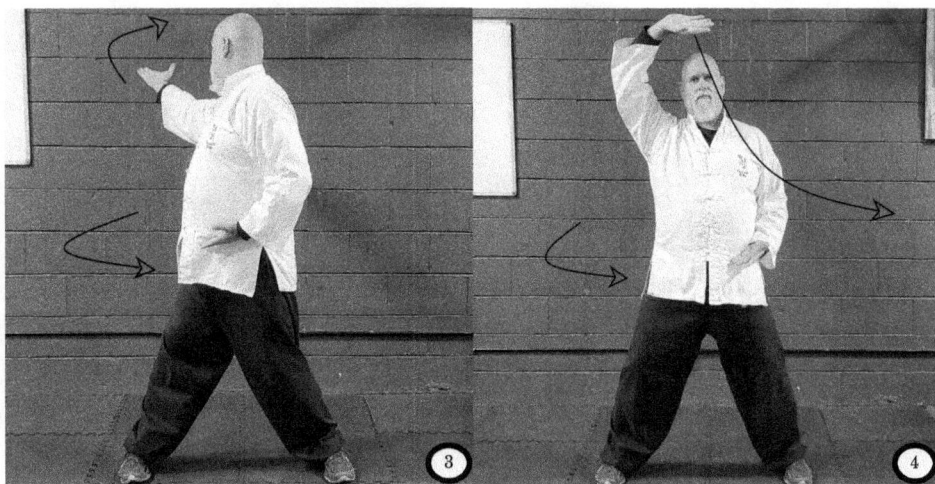

5. Bring your right hand down while rotating your arm to the right keeping your palm facing up, as your hips turn to the left. **6.** Continue to spiral that arm down and back while turning your hips to the right. **7.** Finish by bringing your right arm forward and your hips turn to the left. Repeat on the other side. The goal of this exercise is to squeeze your fascial planes similar to how you might wring out a wet towel.

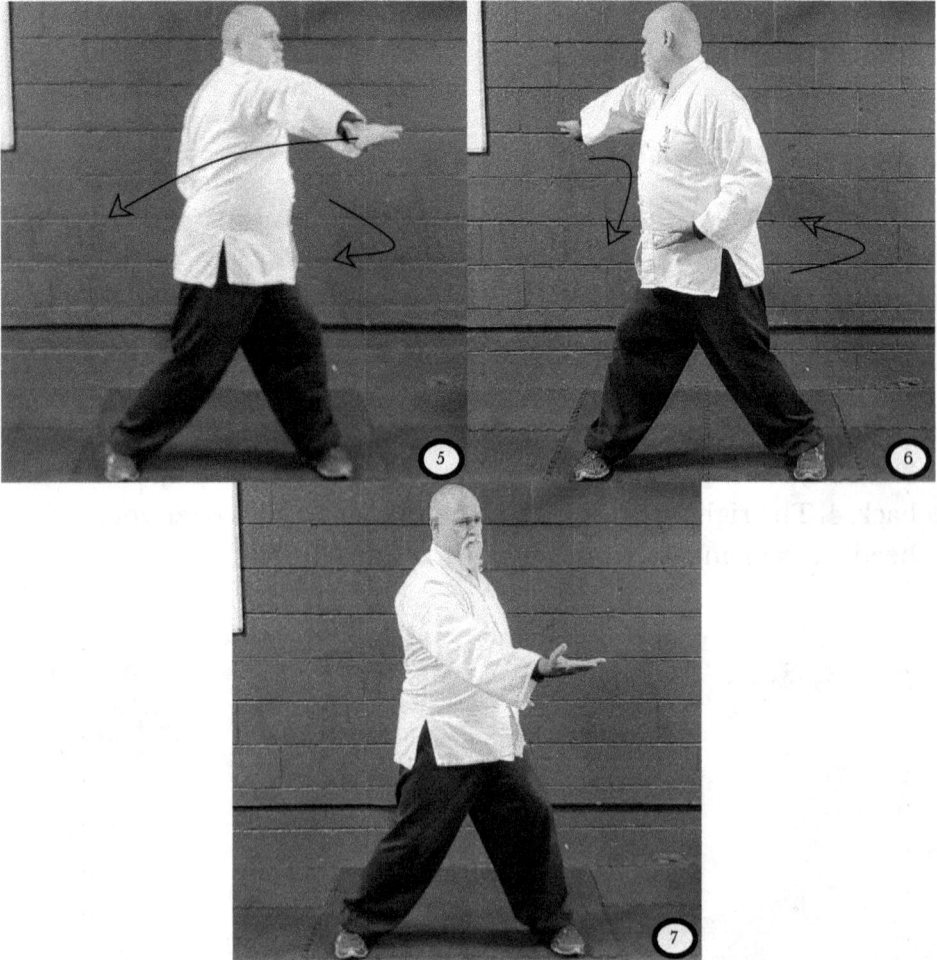

- **Water bucket exercise.** Keep the feet stationary. Bend the knees and rotate the hips to keep the knees and the toes aligned and facing forward. 1. Imagine that you are holding two five-gallon buckets. **2**. Fill the imaginary bucket on the right with water. Let your body shift to the right to accommodate the weight. **3**. Move the water from the right bucket to the left bucket shifting the weight accordingly. The side you are sinking to should feel both heavy and connected. This exercise must be done slowly. Repeat by alternating sides.

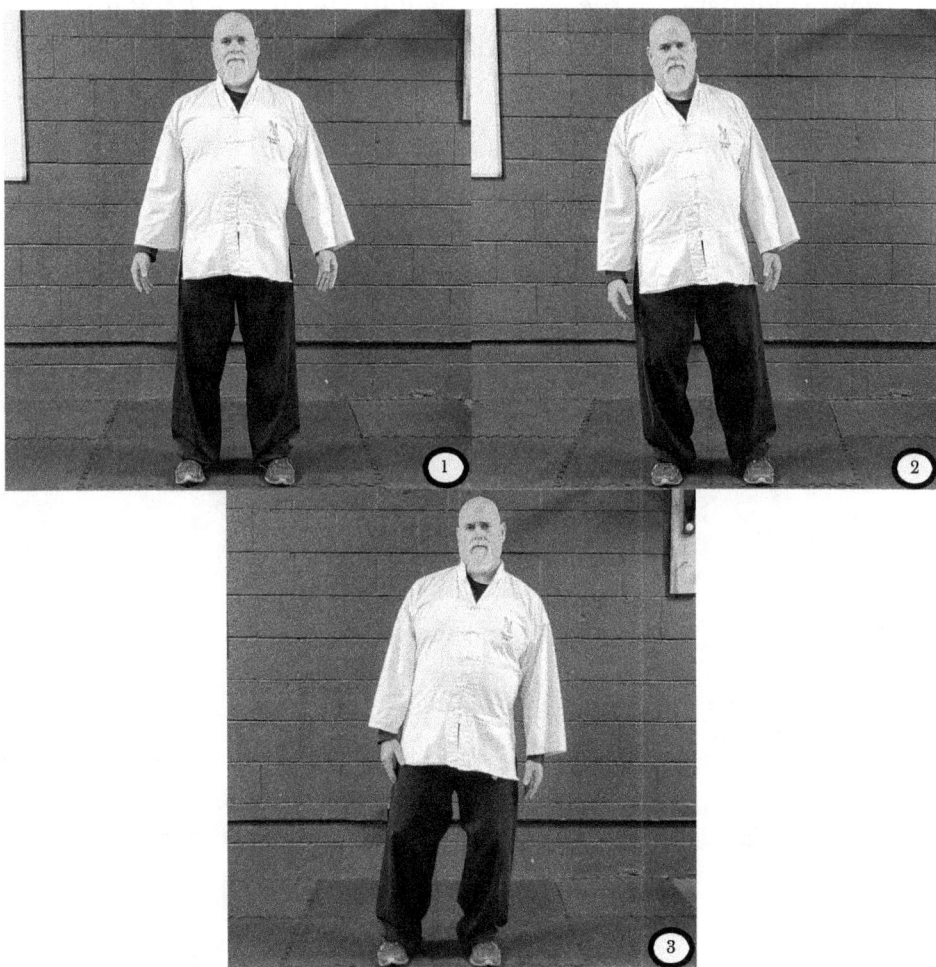

- **Listening drill**. <u>Student One</u> stands in front of <u>Student Two</u> and gently pushes on the following parts of their partner's body— jaw, forehead, occiput, chest, front of shoulder, back of shoulder, side of shoulder, upper back, abdomen, front of hip, side of hip. <u>Student Two</u> practices not resisting the push and moving with the force.

- **Bag drill—sticking. 1**. Adopt a left leg forward 60/40 stance facing the heavy bag. Place the palm of your right hand on the bag and shift forward pushing into it to get the bag in motion. **2**. Keep your right hand on the bag, letting it move you back and forth. As the back come back let it shift your weight onto your back leg. As the bag swings forward follow along with it by shifting your weight forward. Don't add or remove any force to the bag after setting it in motion.

  Also, do this drill with the back of your hand and forearm (not shown).

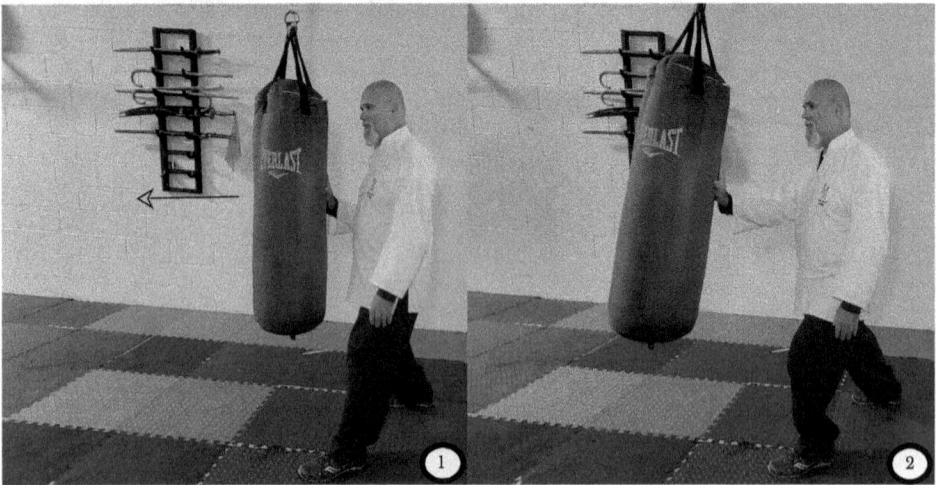

- **Bag drill—wardoff.** Adopt a 60/40 stance facing the heavy bag. Place your lead forearm on the bag. Push the bag to get it in motion. Practice bouncing the bag away. Perform this both while the bag is in the middle of its return arc and at the end of its return arc.

- **Wardoff partner drill against a punch.** Practice using wardoff defensively against a punch by deflecting the energy upwards, outwards, and downwards. Also, practice by entering both to the inside and the outside.

- **Partner shoulder push drill. 1.** Student One starts with their hands on the front of both of Student Two's shoulders. Student One pushes Student Two back until their weight is settled over their back foot in a 60/40 stance. **2.** Student Two then raises their hands to the inside of Student One's elbows with the intention of slightly dislodging their hands and interrupting the force of the push. **3.** Once this is done, Student Two will move their hands forward and attempt to push Student One's shoulders in the same fashion. **4.** When Student One moves into position to return the push to keep the cycle going, they will drop their hands, move them in circles going outside to inside reestablishing their hand position to the inside of their partner's elbows. Repeat.

- Partner shoulder push drill

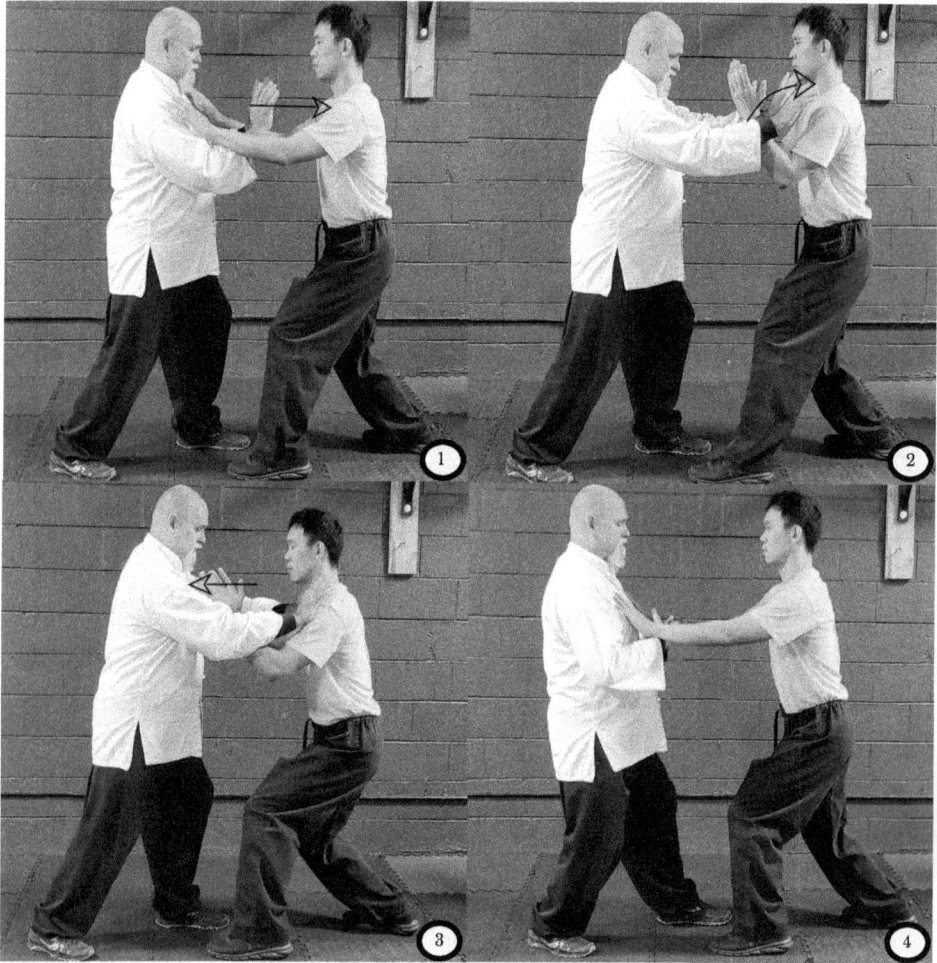

- **Partner shoulder push drill with splitting.** Perform as described above but at the end of the push, the partner being pushed will turn their waist and hips slightly in the direction of their back leg, essentially splitting the energy of their partner's push.

Energetic Skills

Drills intended to improve your sensitivity to *qi* can be more challenging than physical skill development, but they are equally important.

- **Energy drawing.** <u>Student One</u> faces away from <u>Student Two</u>. <u>Student Two</u> focuses *qi* into the index finger and traces out a letter on <u>Student One's</u> back without touching them. <u>Student One</u> identifies the letter being drawn.

- **Fire focusing drill.** This is a solo drill. Stand in a small horse stance with hands approximately 10 inches apart. Close your eyes and emit *qi* from one hand to the other. Imagine you are holding a fire. See if you can feel an increase in temperature.

- **Fire focusing partner drill.** Same as the above drill but now your partner puts their hand in between your hands.

- **Push/pull.** This drill requires three students. <u>Student One</u> is the target, their job is to stand and relax. <u>Student Two</u> is the pusher. Their job is to get into a 60/40 stance behind <u>Student One</u>, and using a technique like push, they try to emit *qi* through their hands and get <u>Student One</u> to gently rock back and forth without touching them. <u>Student Three</u> is the objective observer watching to see if there is movement.

- ***Qi* sensitivity drill.** Start with your hands 24"-36" apart. Slowly bring them together while emitting *qi* from PC-8 until you can feel the *qi* sensation in the palm of your other hand. A variation of this is to point one finger at the other open palm and emit *qi*.

The Simplified Form (24-Move)

24-Move Simplified or "Short Form"

1. Commence Tai Chi

2. Parting the Wild Horses Mane

3. White Stork Spreads Wings

4. Brush Knee

5. Play the Pei Pa

6. Step Back and Repulse Monkey

7. Grasp Sparrow's Tail – Left

8. Grasp Sparrow's Tail – Right

9. Single Whip

10. Wave Hands Like Clouds

11. Single Whip

12. High Pat on Horse

13. Kick Right

14. Box Tiger at Ears

15. Kick Left

16. Snake Creeps Low/Golden Cock Stands on One Leg – Left

17. Snake Creeps Low/Golden Cock Stands on One Leg – Right

18. Fair Lady Works the Shuttles

19. Push Needle to Sea Bottom

20. Fan Through Back

21. Step Up, Deflect, Parry, and Punch

22. Apparent Withdrawal

23. Cross Hands

24. End Tai Chi

Attention. 1. Feet together, facing 12 o'clock. Knees slightly bent. Head erect, eyes facing forward. Hands held at sides. Drop the tension out of your shoulders. Chest is slightly concave. Clear your mind of any stray thoughts. **2.** When you are ready to begin move your hands to cover your *tan tien*.

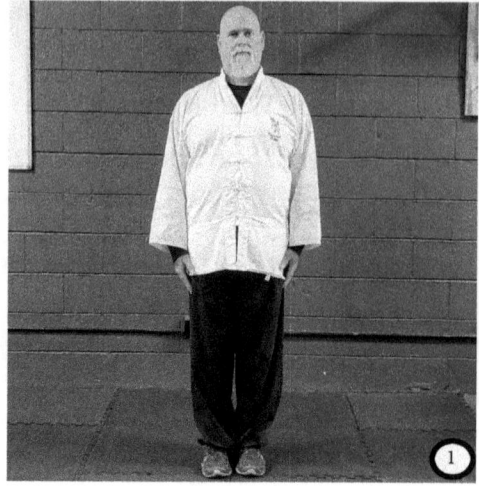

Commence Tai Chi. 3. Shift your weight to the right leg, lift up your left foot starting with the heel, and step to the left. Toes go first then put the heel down. You are stepping into a small horse stance. Keep both knees slightly bent. **4.** Drop hands to sides.

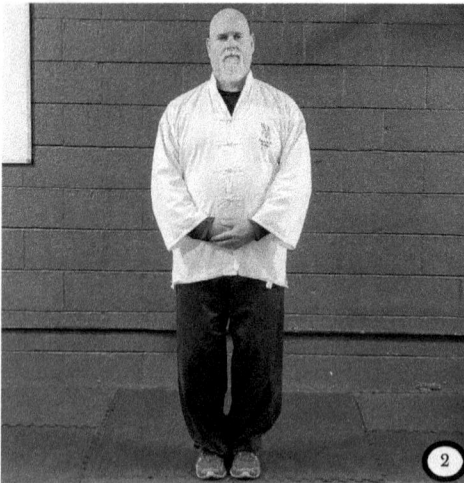
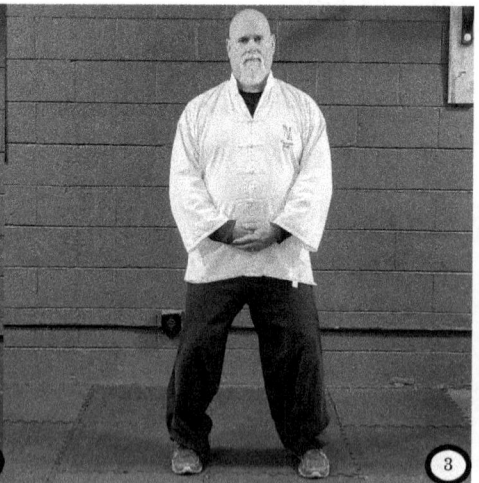

5. Hands float up until they are in front of your shoulders, elbows slightly bent and palms face down. 6. Bring your hands back into your chest and push down, fingers face forwards. 7. End with palms flat and slight tension on the back of your wrists.

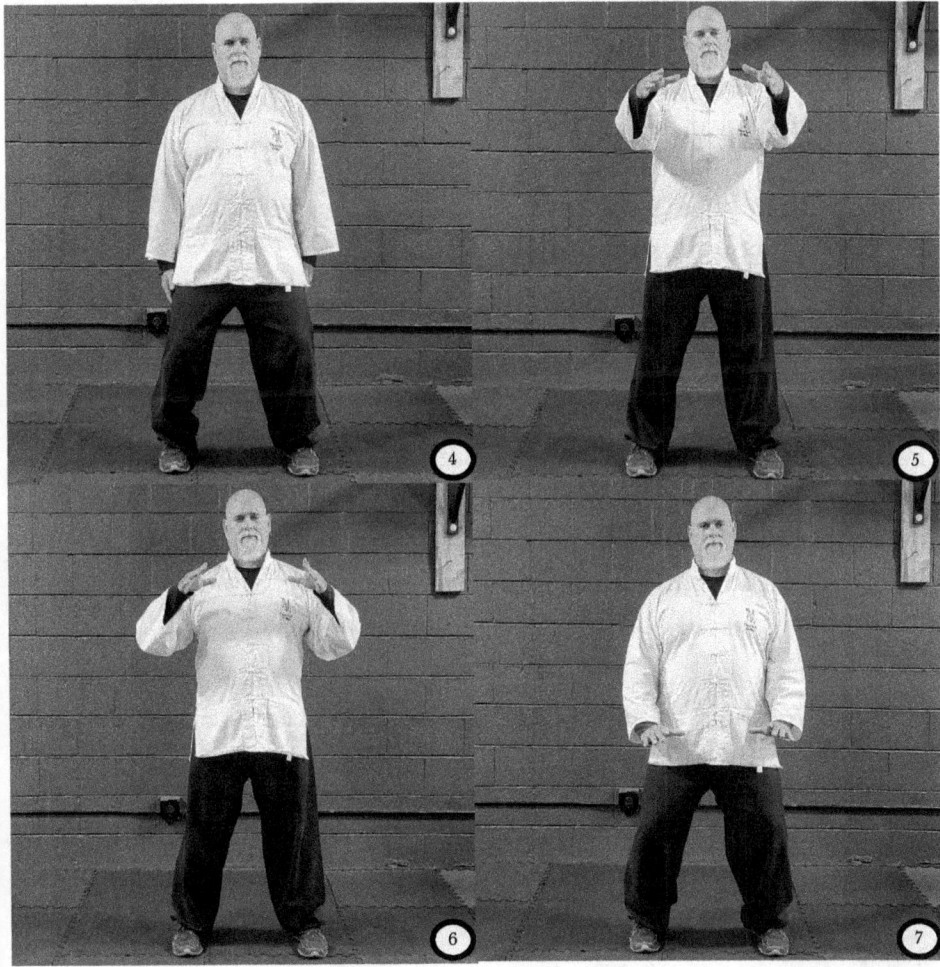

Hold Right Ball. 8. Turn your hips to the right bringing your right hand back and your left hand forward. Right hand circles back and up, ending palm down at your right shoulder. Left hand circles in, ending at your left hip, palm up. As your hands are moving turn your hips to the left ending in a cat stance facing 9 o'clock. Right knee is slightly bent. When you finish this move your right foot, hips, and shoulders are facing 10:30, and your left foot and head are facing 9 o'clock. Hold Right Ball is not a separate move in the form but it is an often used transition.

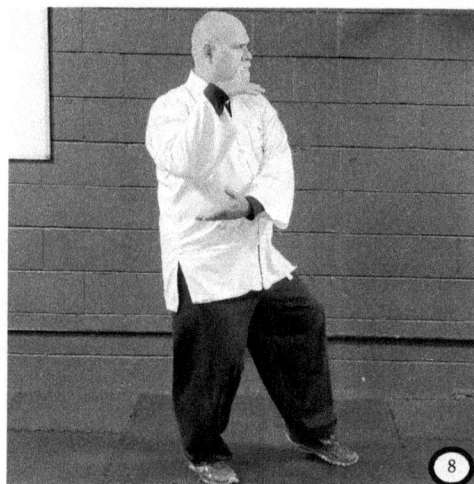

Parting the Wild Horse's Mane. 9. Step forward with your left foot into a 60/40 stance. Your left hand moves up and out, elbow is down. Your hand stops in front of your left shoulder, fingers at eye level. Your right hand moves down approximately one fists distance in front of your hip. Elbow is straight but not locked.

Parting the Wild Horses Mane (side view)   Parting the Wild Horses Mane (front view)

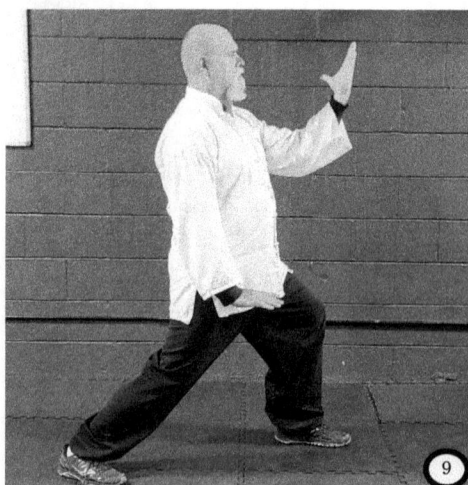

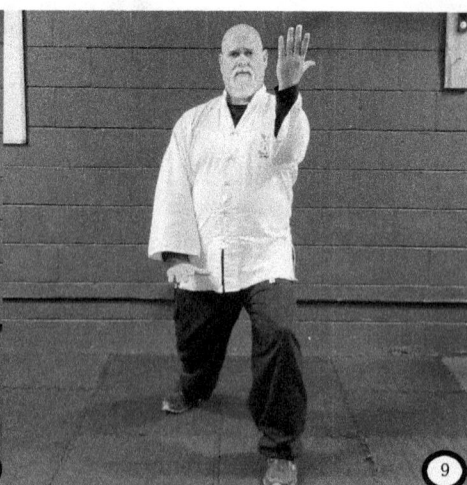

128

Parting the Wild Horse's Mane.
10-13. Repeat a total of three times, alternating left, right, and left, moving towards 9 o'clock You will hold a right or left ball as you transition into the next Parting the Wild Horse's Mane each time.

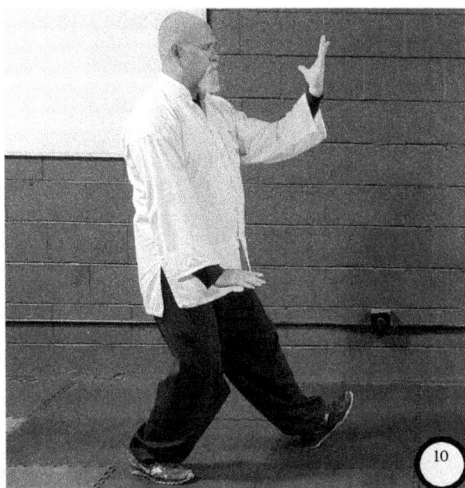

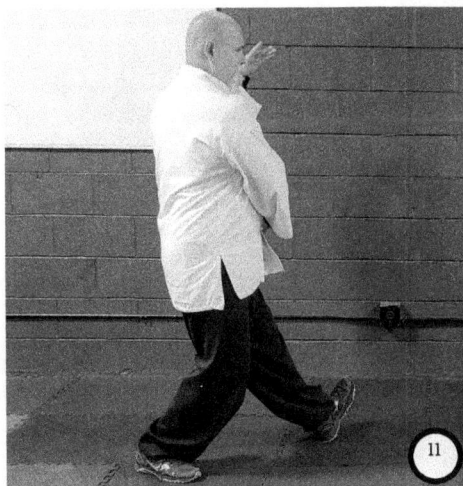

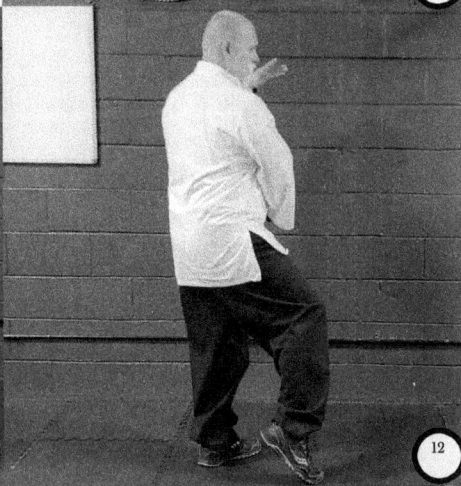

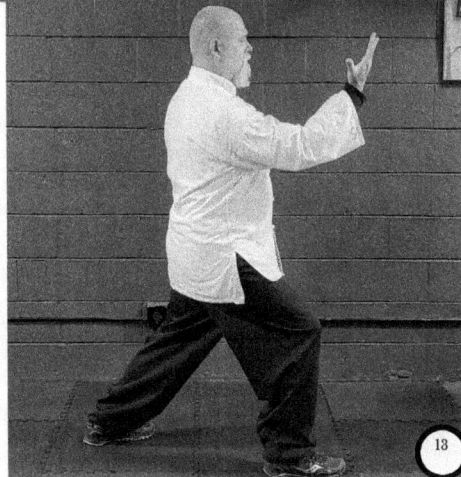

Parting the Wild Horse's Mane Applied. 1. Student Two attacks Student One with a right punch. Student One intercepts the punch to the outside, with his right hand while simultaneously chambering his left hand for a counterattack. **2.** Student One turns his hips to the right, grabs Student Two's hand at the wrist pulling him forward and down and brings his left arm to the front of Student Two's chest. **3.** Student One steps forward with his left foot to the outside of Student Two's right foot. This puts his hands and body into position to either strike Student Two's neck with his left ridge hand, throw Student Two over his left leg, or apply a joint lock to Student Two's right elbow.

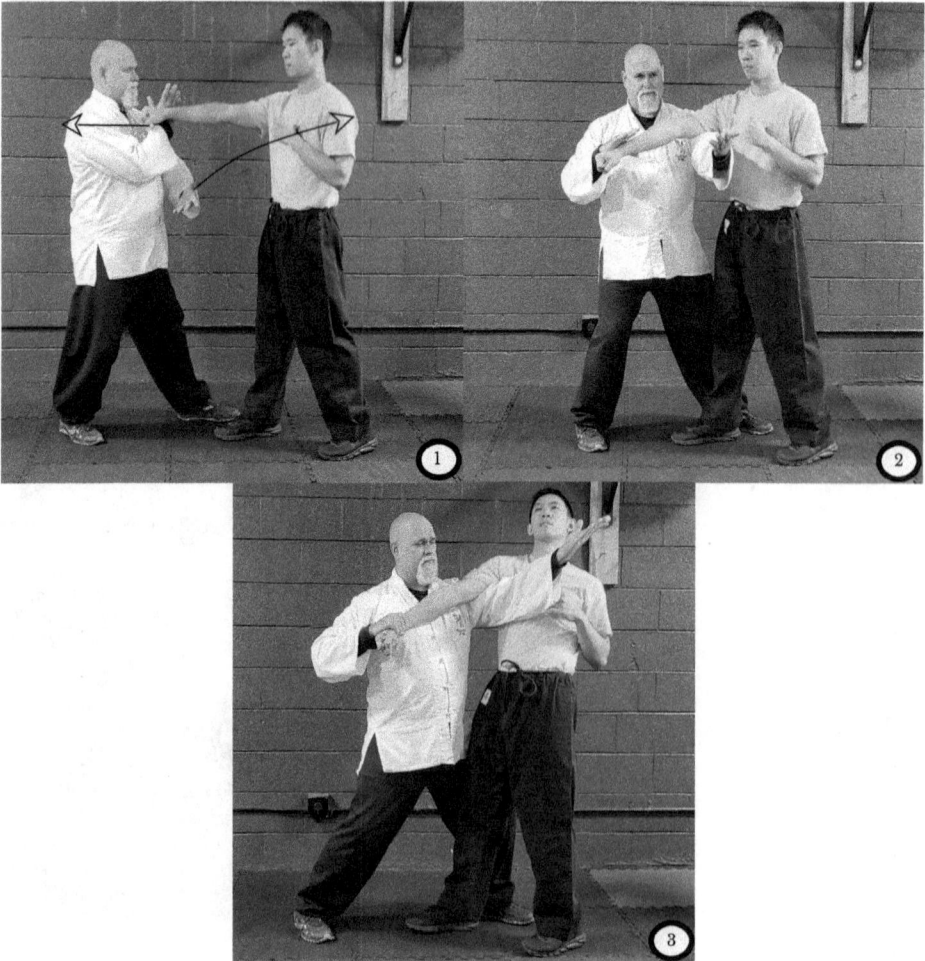

White Stork Spreads Wings. 14. From the previous move, take a half step forward with your right foot ending in a left foot forward cat stance facing 9 o'clock. Your right hand moves up, stopping just above your head while your left hand simultaneously moves down towards your left hip. Extend but don't lock your left arm, left palm is facing the ground fingers face forwards. Shift your hands to the left, then shift them to the right, ending with chambering your right hand near your right ear.

White Stork Spreads Wings (front view)

White Stork Spreads Wings (side view)

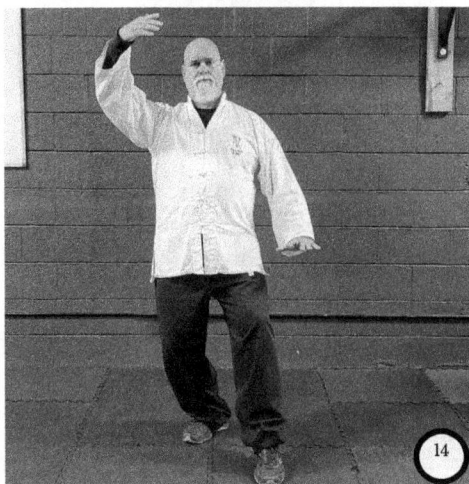

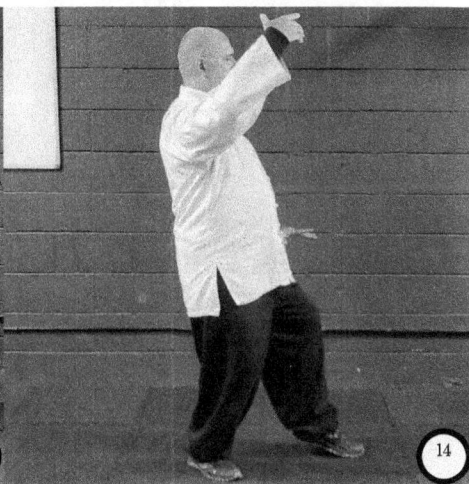

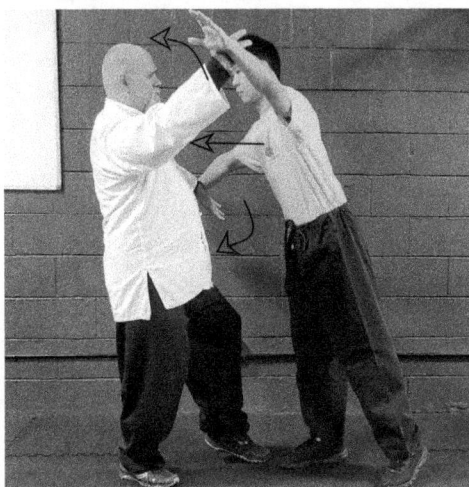

White Stork Spreads Wings Applied. Student Two attacks Student One with a two hand push from the front. Student One fades the attack by moving into a right leg back cat stance while simultaneously sweeping his left arm out and down and his right arm up and out (Splitting *jing*). This disrupts Student Two's attack while at the same time setting Student One up for a left front kick to Student Two's groin.

Brush Knee and Twist Step. 15. From Hold Right Ball. **16.** Step forward with your left foot into a 60/40 stance towards 9 o'clock pushing forward with your right palm as you do so. Your left hand sweeps down toward your left hip, ending palm down and fingers facing forward, approximately one fist away from your hip. **17-19.** Repeat two more times alternating left and right, moving towards 9 o'clock.

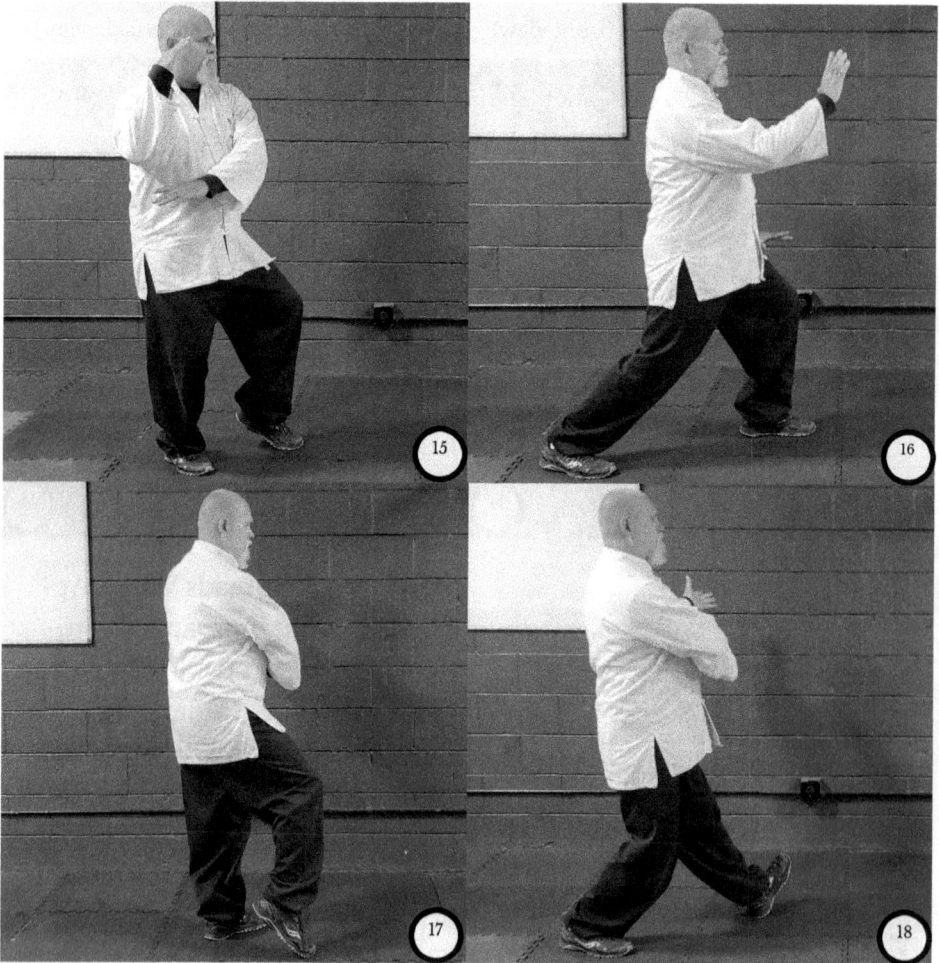

Brush Knee and Twist Step (side view)   Brush Knee and Twist Step (front view)

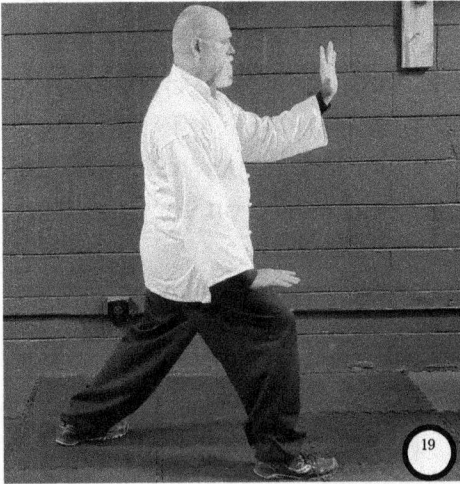

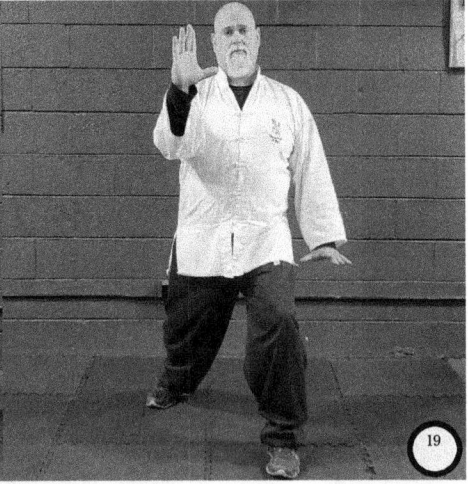

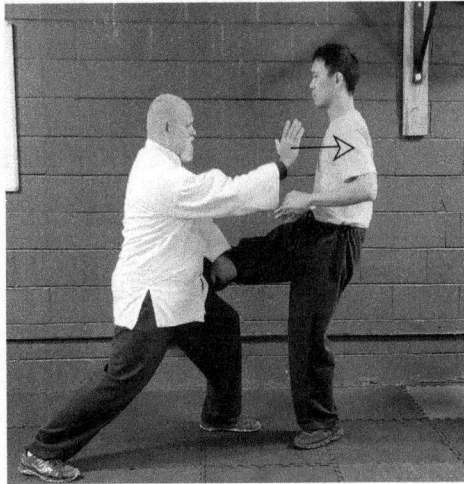

Brush Knee and Twist Step Applied. <u>Student Two</u> kicks at <u>Student One</u>. <u>Student One</u> steps into <u>Student Two</u> with his left foot and simultaneously deflects the kick to the left with his left hand and counterattacks with a right knifehand chop to the chest.

Play the Peipa. 20. From the previous move take a half step forward to 9 o'clock with your right foot ending in a cat stance with your left toes up. Left hand circles up ending with your left hand in front of your left shoulder, fingers at eye level. Your right hand circles in, ending palm facing in, at the level of your left elbow. When your arms complete their movements they should be separated approximately one fists distance from each other centered on your midline.

Play the Peipa (front view)   **Play the Peipa (side view)**

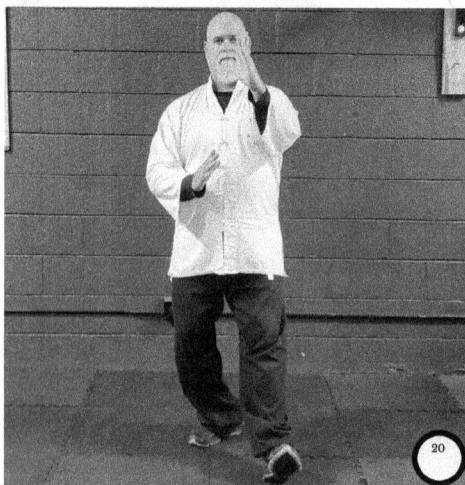

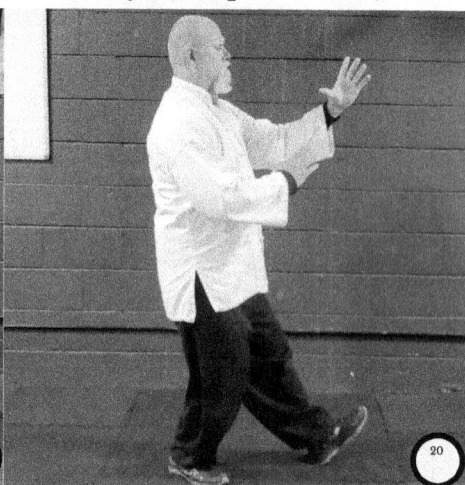

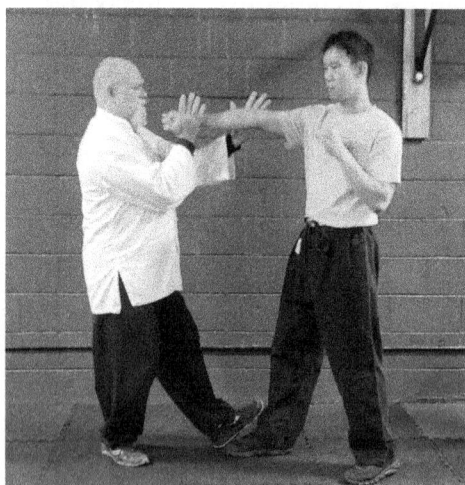

Play the Peipa Applied. Student Two punches Student One. Student One fades backwards ending in a toes up cat stance. The hands move up to intercept the punch, facilitating both a capture and a block. When pressure is applied the block turns into a joint lock. Student One's left foot can trap Student Two's right leg or it can be a front kick.

134

Step Back and Repulse Monkey. 21. From the previous move shift your weight to your right leg, left hand moves up and your right hand moves back. **22.** Lift up your left knee above the level of your waist. Your right arm swings down and back ending palm up at the level of your right shoulder and your left arm goes forward and up. **23.** Step back towards 3 o'clock with your left foot leading with your toes. **24.** At the same time as you step back with your left leg push forward with your right palm and retract your left hand. Settle into a 60/40 stance with your right hand forward and your left hand, palm up, in front of your *tan tien*. Repeat three more times alternating right, left, right. End by moving into hold right ball, facing 9 o'clock.

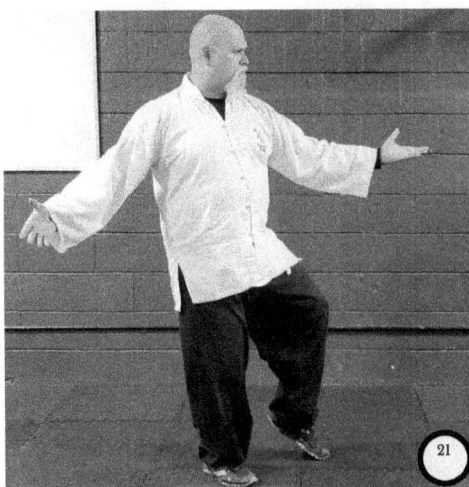

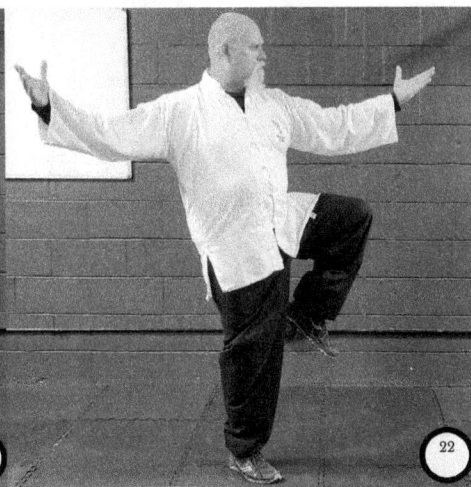

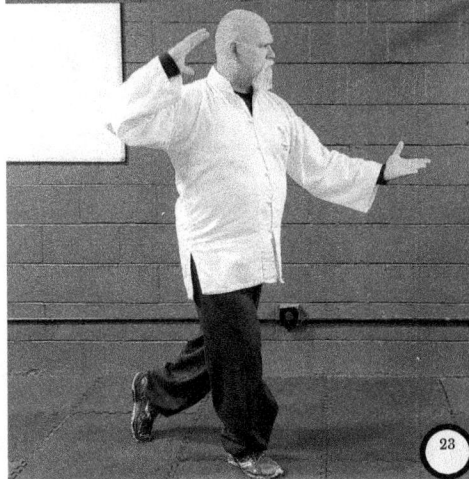

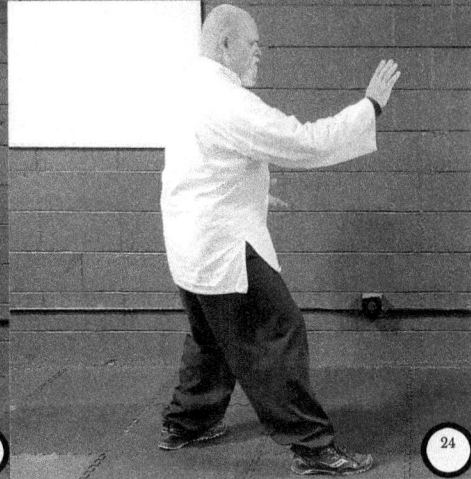

Step Back and Repulse Monkey Applied. 1. <u>Student Two</u> grabs <u>Student One's</u> left wrist with his left hand. **2.** <u>Student One</u> shifts his weight back onto his right foot simultaneously circling his left hand in and up and he raises his left knee. (If <u>Student Two</u> is close enough, this rising knee can be used to strike the groin as part of <u>Student One's</u> counterattack).

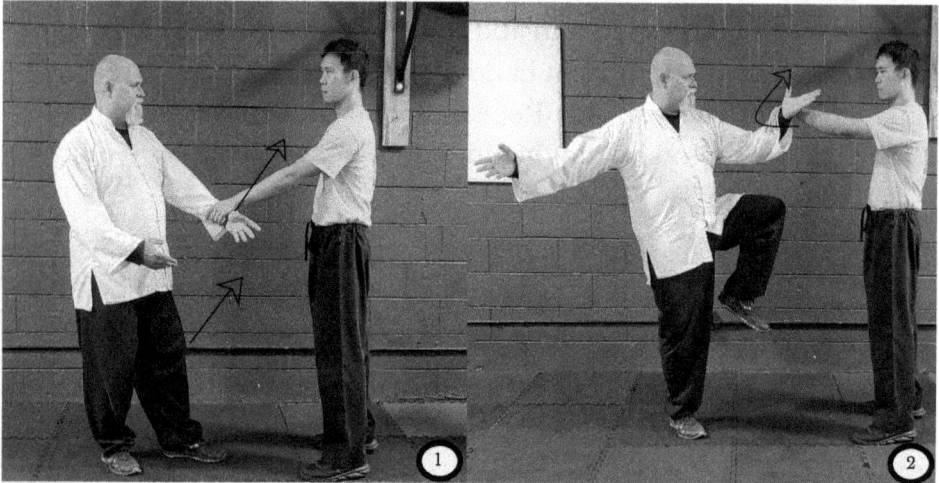

3. <u>Student One</u> counter-grabs <u>Student Two's</u> left wrist and chambers his right hand above the shoulder in preparation for the counterattack. **4.** <u>Student One</u> steps backwards with his left leg, pulling <u>Student One</u> forward and down, off-balancing him. <u>Student One</u> then brings his right hand down for an arm bar.

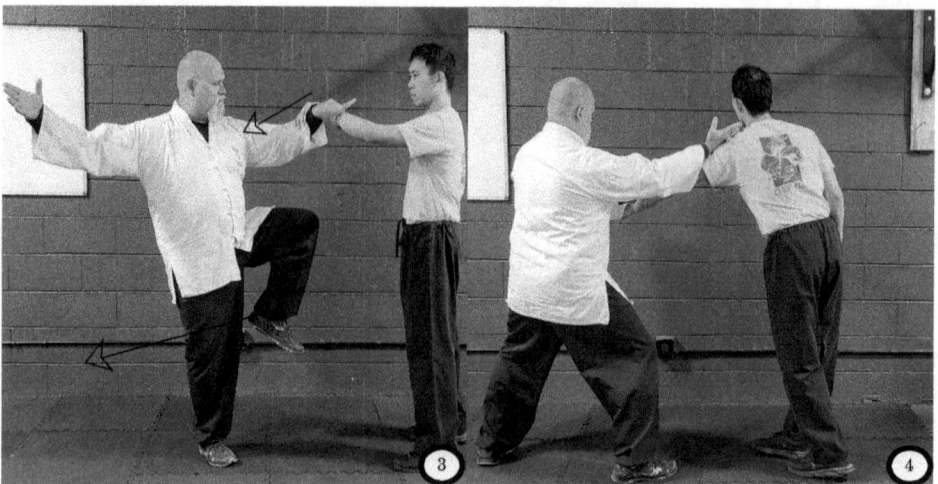

Grasp Sparrows Tail. 25. From Hold Right Ball, step forward to 9 o'clock ending in a 60/40 stance with your left foot forward. **26**. Both arms move forward, your left hand will stop at the level of your left shoulder palm facing in, your right hand will be at the level of your left elbow. **27**. Keeping the arms up and in the same general position, rotate both hands approximately 180 degrees. You will finish with your left palm facing out and your right palm facing in. **28**. Shift your weight to your right leg turning your hips to the right. Allow your arms to swing down and to the right. Your right arm will end at approximately the level of your right shoulder, your left hand will be at the level of your right elbow.

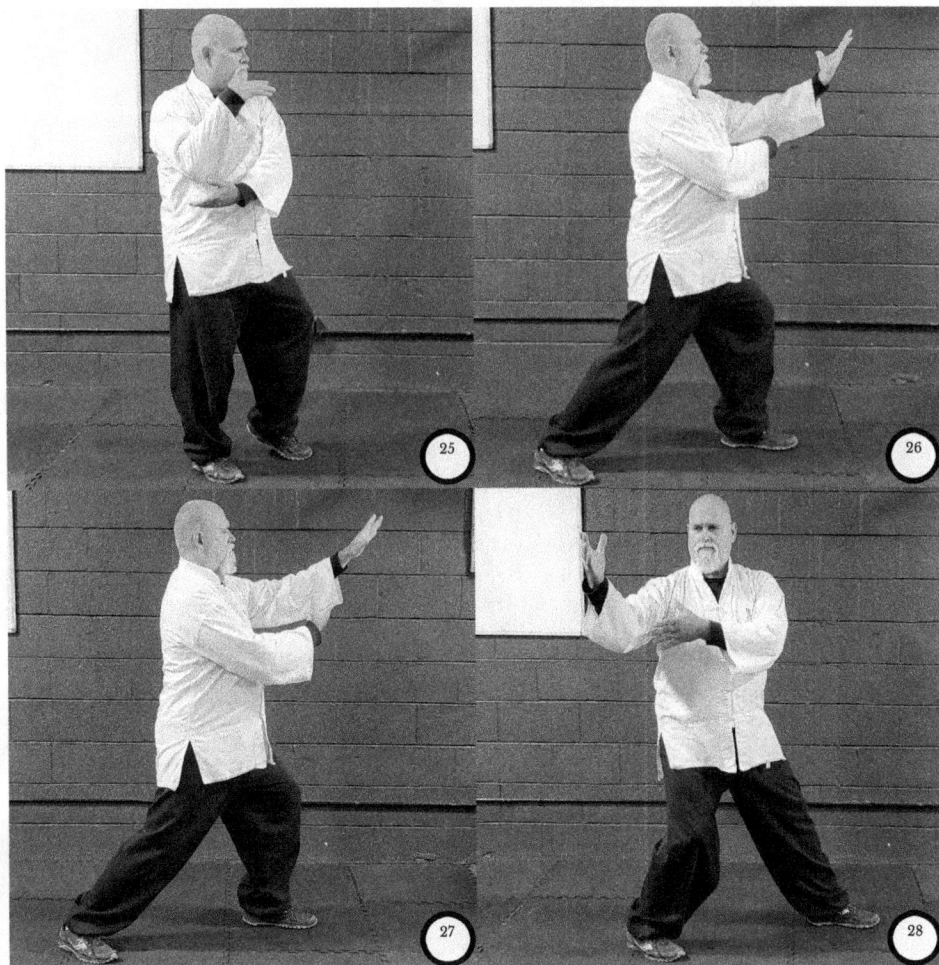

29. Turn your hips to the left, with your left arm horizontal and your right hand at the level of your left wrist, but not touching. Shift your weight to your left leg in a 60/40 stance. This is known as "wardoff". **30.** Cross your right hand over your left hand at the wrist, your weight is still forward. **31.** Separate hands, your left hand moves to the left and your right hand moves to the right. **32.** Bring the backs of both hands backwards towards the chest, as you shift your weight to your right leg.

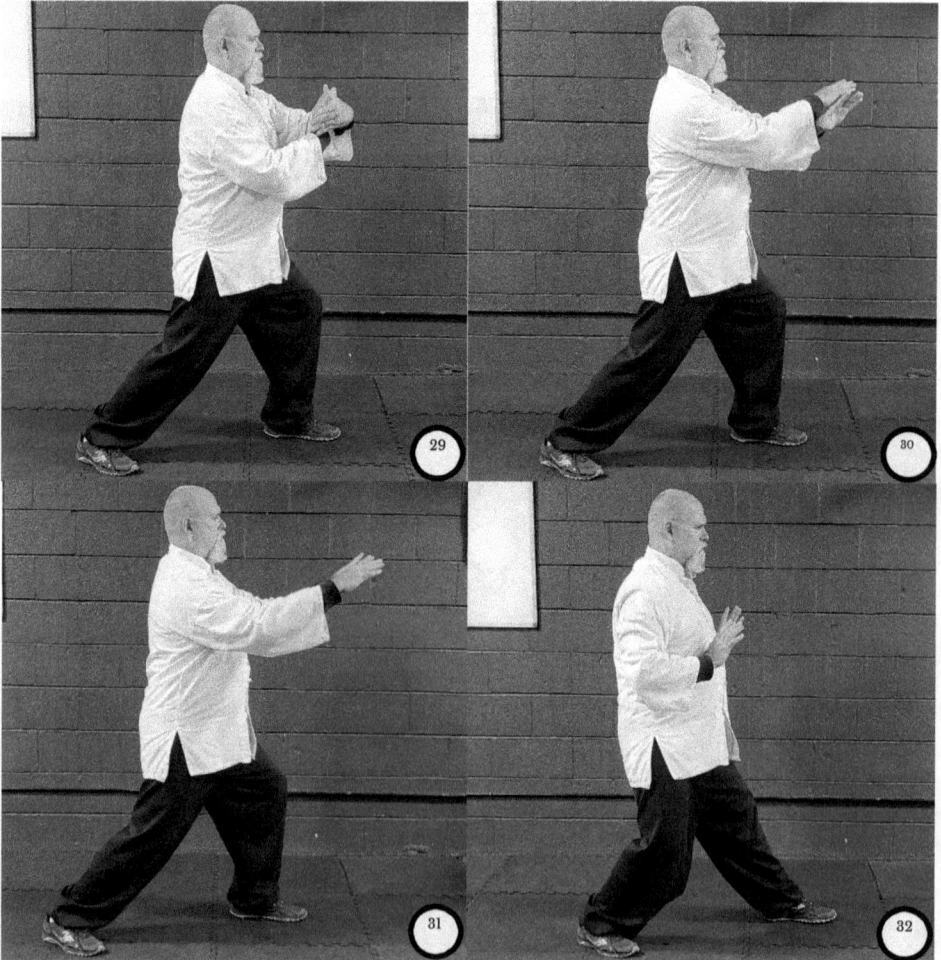

33. Both hands continue their circular motion dropping to the level of your *tan tien*. Your weight is over your back leg. **34.** Push both hands forward and up, palms facing forward, fingers up as you shift forward into a 60/40 stance with your weight on your left foot. Repeat on the right side.

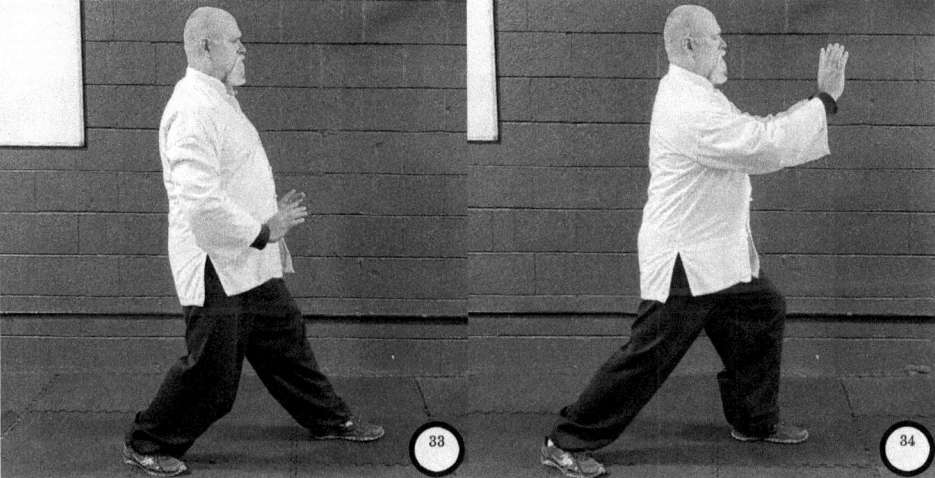

Single Whip. 35. From the end of the previous move, rock back putting your weight onto your left foot. Turn your hips to the left both arms are extended forward. Allow your right foot to turn to the left on the heel. Your hands will move in a circle to the left, then bring them into the chest. Extend your right hand towards 12 o'clock in a crane beak. You will be in a cat stance briefly. Step into a 60/40 stance towards 9 o'clock and push forward with your left hand.

Single Whip (side view)   Single Whip (front view)

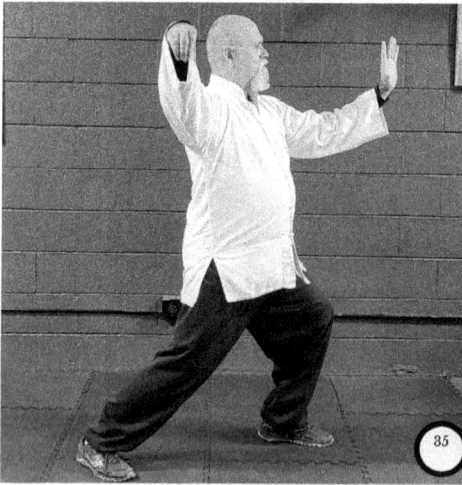

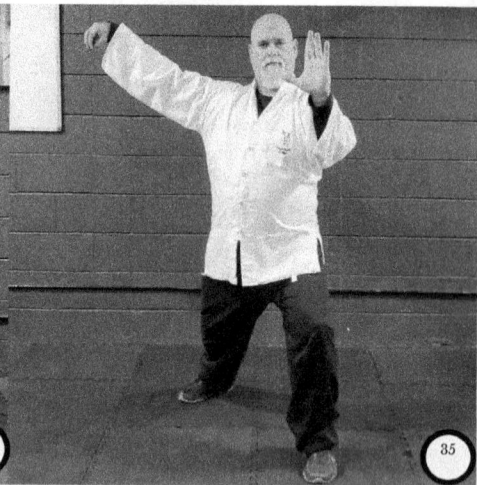

Wave Hands Like Clouds. 36. Shift your weight to your right foot, left toes lift up. Turn your hips to the right opening up your right hand as you do. Your left foot turns in 90 degrees to the right on the heel. Right hand circles to the right at the level of your head palm facing out while your left hand drops, palm in, at the level of your *tan tien*. Hands continue their circular motion and your hips continue turning to the right until they are facing 12 o'clock.

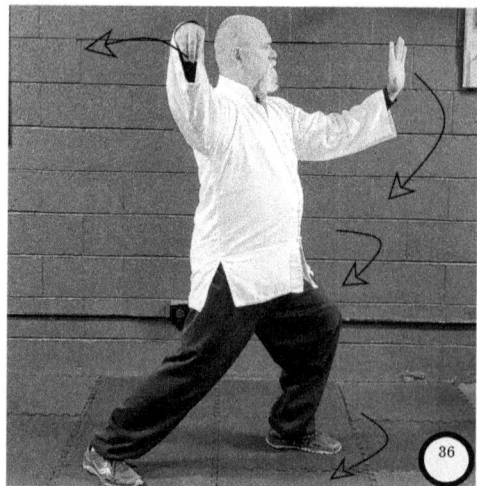

37. Shift your weight to your right foot, bring your arms to the right. Hands and hips continue to turn to the right until both hands are at shoulder level, your right hand is extended and your left hand is close to your body. **38**. Shift your weight to the center by turning your hips to the left, your left hand is at the level of your face, your right hand is in front of your *tan tien*.

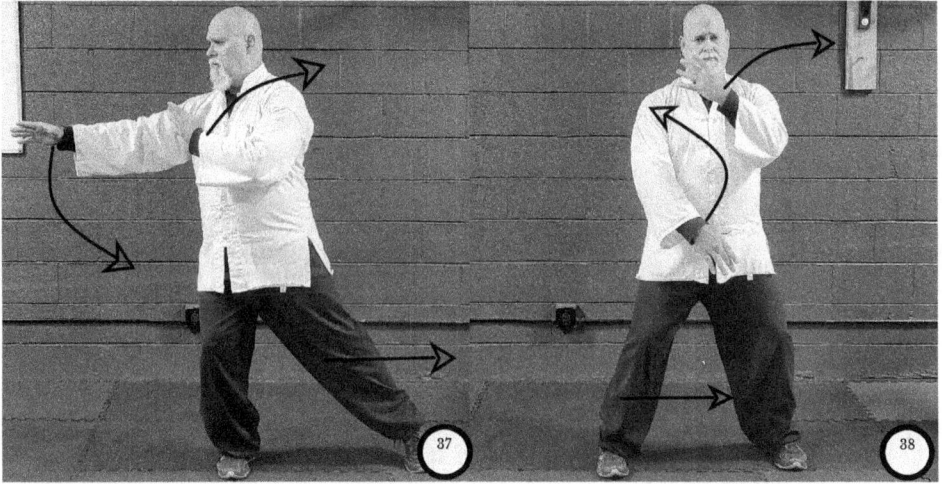

39. Continue to circle both hands to the left, shift weight to your left foot as your hips turn to the left. Lift your right heel in preparation to the step to the left side. **40**. Weight comes back to the center as you step to the left with your right foot, bringing both feet together.

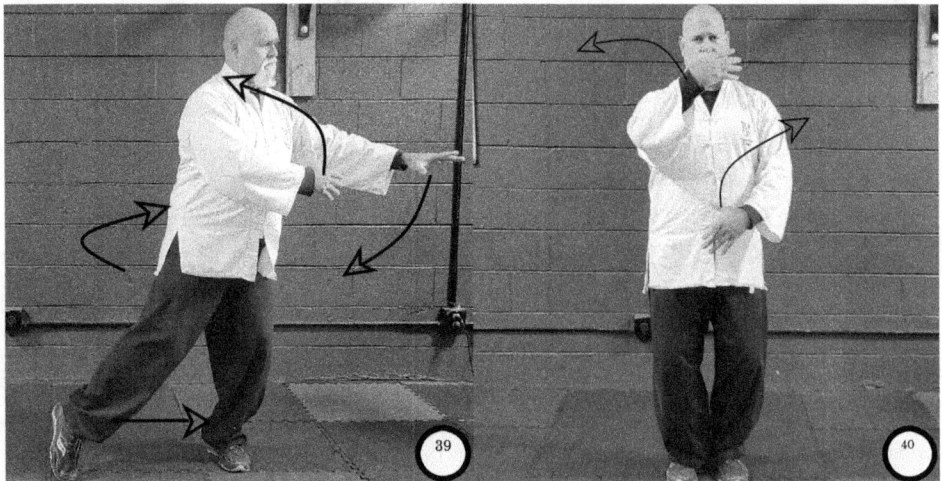

41-43. Continue this process of side stepping to the left for a total of three times. Let the motion of your hips turning side-to-side move your arms from left to right, let gravity move your arms down, and let momentum lift your arms up.

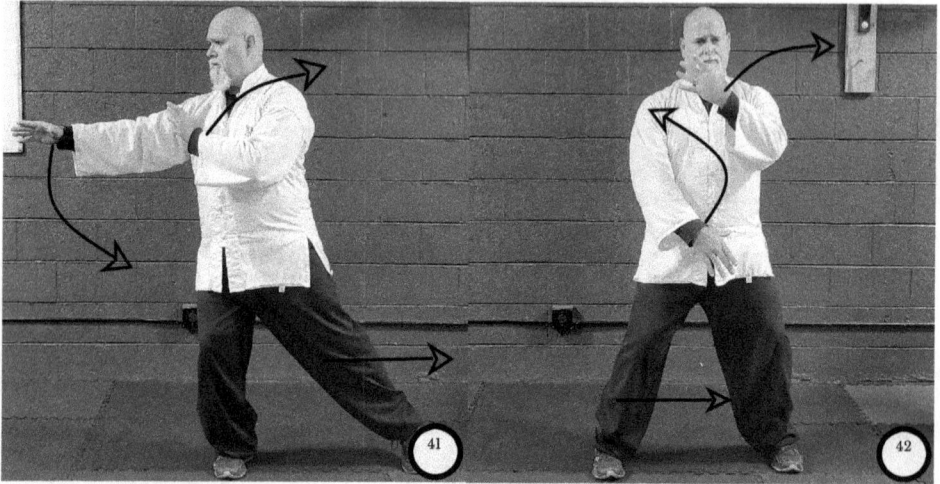

44. When you finish the last <u>Wave Hands Like Clouds</u> step, preset your right foot by turning it to face 10:30, then step with your left foot to 9 o'clock, settling into a 60/40 stance. Right hand goes into crane beak, left hand pushes forward. You will end in <u>Single Whip</u>, with your left foot forward, facing 9 o'clock.

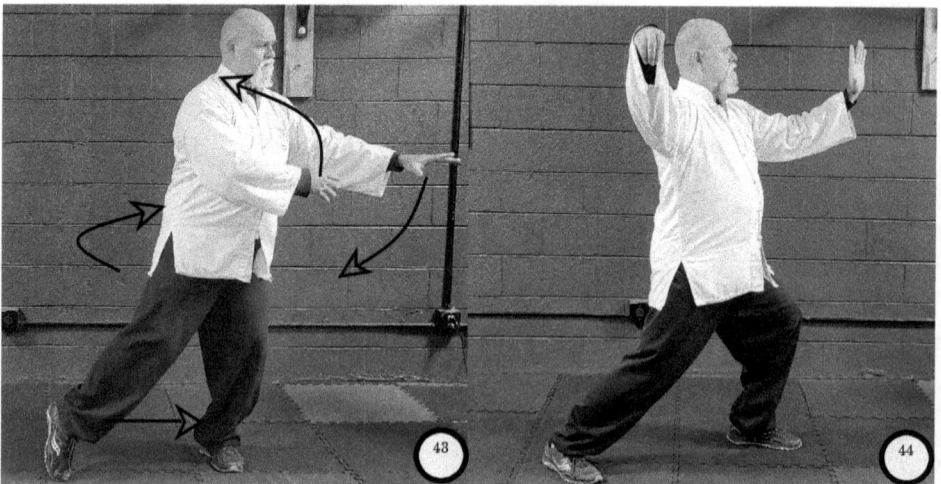

High Pat on Horse. 45. From previous move take a half step forward with your right foot ending in a right leg back cat stance. Your left hand moves palm up, approximately one fists distance in front of your *tan tien*. Simultaneously your right hand pushes forward, palm out, ending at about the level of your face. Both of your hands are aligned with your midline.

High Pat on Horse (side view)   High Pat on Horse (front view)

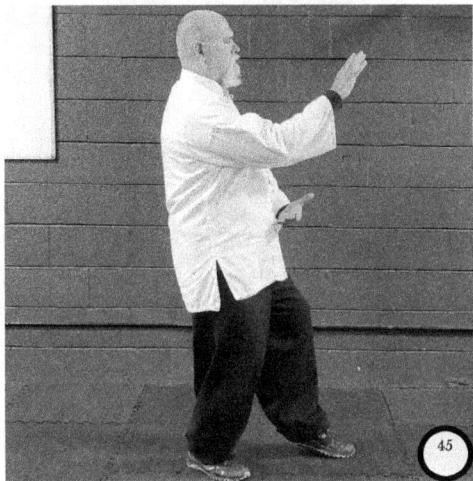

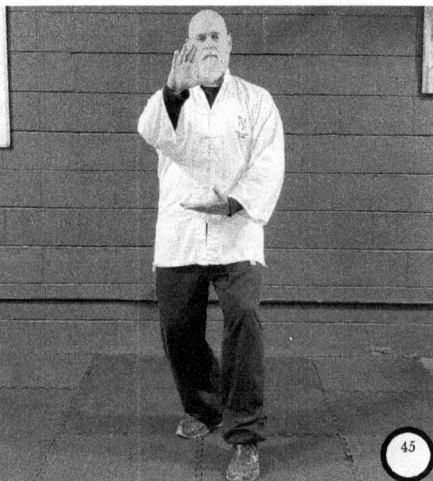

Kick Right/Left. 46. Step to the left with your left foot, arms circle out to the sides, ending crossed at the wrists with your right hand on the outside. Bring your right leg up into a crane stance with your right knee above the level of your waist. Right hand pushes to 9 o'clock, left hand pushes to 6 o'clock, and execute a right heel kick to 9 o'clock. Perform <u>Box Tiger as Ears</u>, then turn to the left and <u>Kick Left</u> by repeating the above moves on the left side, facing to 3 o'clock.

Kick Right (front view)

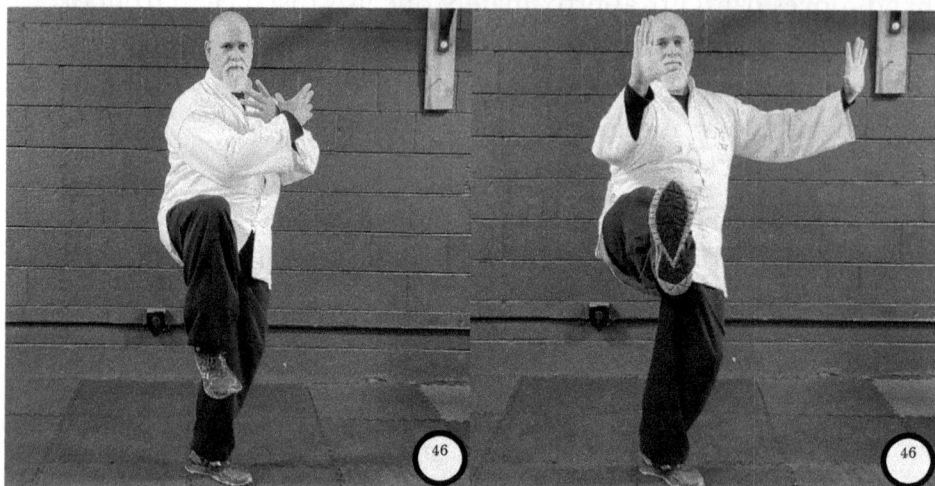

Kick Right (side view)

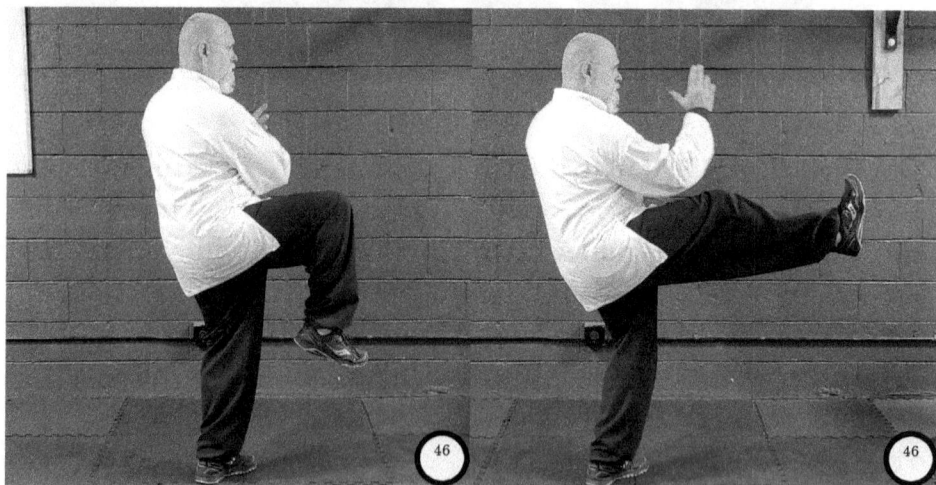

Box Tiger at Ears. 47. From the end of <u>Kick Right</u>, rechamber your right leg and step forward to 9 o'clock into a 60/40 stance. Hands chamber into tai chi fists, palms down, at your waist. As you shift your weight forward onto your right toes, strike forward and up hitting with your first two knuckles at about the level of your head. <u>Box Tiger at Ears</u> is followed by <u>Kick Left</u>.

Box Tiger at Ears (front view)   **Box Tiger at Ears (side view)**

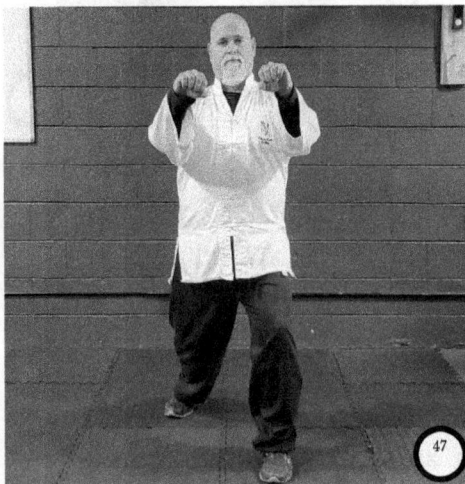

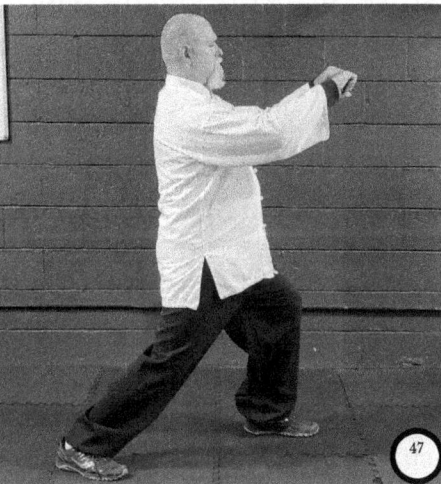

Snake Creeps Low. 48. Right hand moves to 6 o'clock in a crane beak with your fingertips at the level of the top of your shoulder. Knife hand thrust with your left hand along the inside of your left leg. Bend your right knee as you step forward with your left foot into a snake creeps low stance.

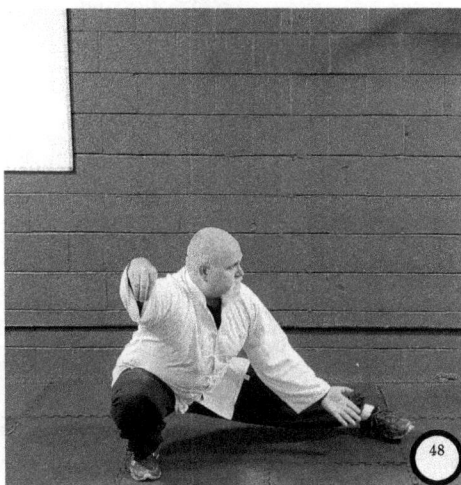

49. Stand upright and shift your weight to your left foot in a 60/40 stance. Your right hand circles down and back striking low in a crane beak, your left hand pushes forward, palm out. As you settle into your stance your hips turn to the left to facilitate the palm strike. Snake Creeps Low is followed by Golden Cock Stands on One Leg. Repeat on both sides.

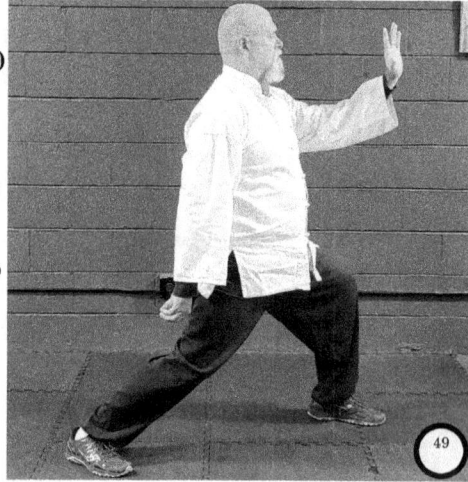

Kick Right and Box Tiger at Ears Applied. Student Two punches at Student One. As Student Two steps in to attack, Student One kicks him in the abdomen with the heel of his right foot. Simultaneously, Student One deflects the incoming punch to the left with his left hand and strikes forward with a right knife hand chop. He continues his counter attack by stepping into Student Two with his right foot, chambering both hands at his waist, and striking forward and up with the 2nd MCP joints of both hands to Student Two's temples.

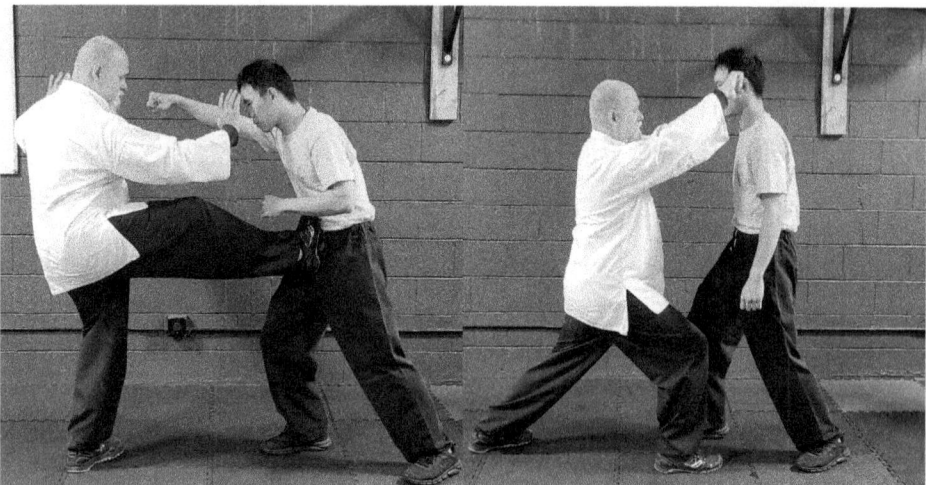

Golden Cock Stands on One Leg. 50. Shift your weight to your right leg by slightly bending your right knee and sinking your weight. Lift your left toes. Open your *kua* on the left side by turning your left foot out 45 degrees to the left. Shift your weight onto your left foot while simultaneously moving into a right leg up crane stance, with your right knee above the level of your waist. Right hand, palm facing in, at the level of your right shoulder. Left hand, palm facing in, at the level of your right elbow. Golden Cock Stands on One Leg is done at the end of Snake Creeps Low. Repeat on both sides.

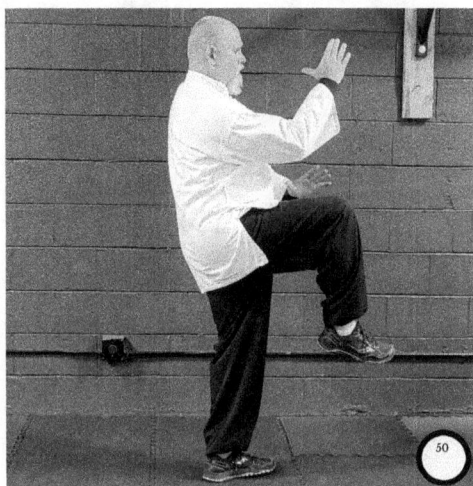

Fair Lady Works the Shuttle. 51. From Golden Cock Stands on One Leg bring your left foot down, both hands move, palms down fingers forward in front of your *tan tien*. Shift your weight to the left and hold left ball. Open your right hip, and step to the right. Shift your weight to the right into a 60/40 stance. Simultaneously your right hand moves up, palm out, thumb faces down and your left hand pushes to the right, thumb up, palm out. Both of your hands are in the same plane. Shift your weight to the right, hold right ball and repeat to the other side.

Fair Lady Works the Shuttle (side view)   Fair Lady Works the Shuttle (front view)

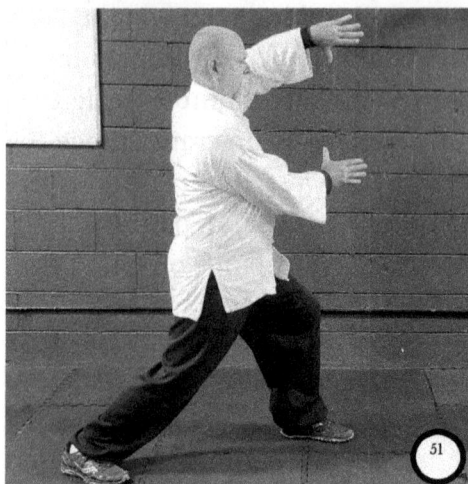

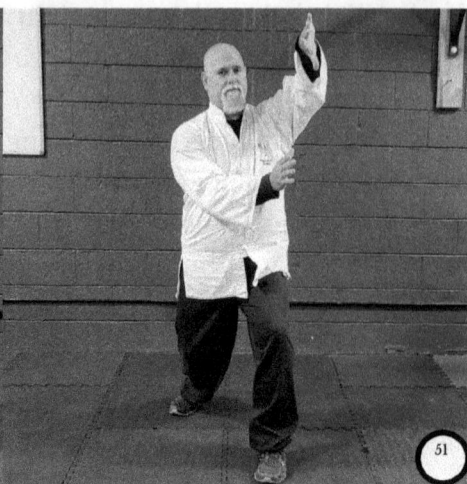

Push Needle to Sea Bottom. 52. Bring both hands down and turn your hips to the right, arms move to the right. Your right hand chambers near your right ear, your left hand moves to the right side of your torso, palm up. Transition into a left foot forward cat stance while your left hand sweeps low to the outside of your left knee and your right knife hand thrusts forward and down. Slightly bend at the waist but keep your back straight.

Push Needle to Sea Bottom (front view)   Push Needle to Sea Bottom (side view)

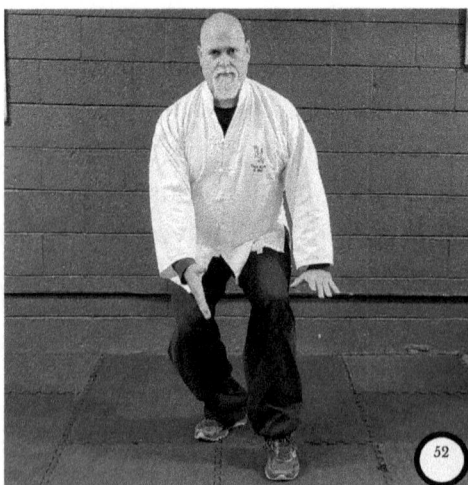

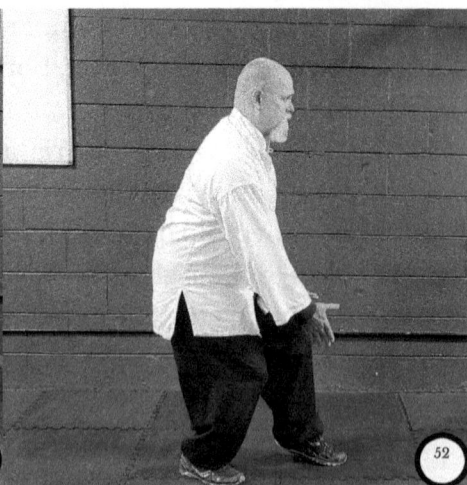

Fan Through Back. 53. Straighten your back and step forward with your left foot into a 60/40 stance to 3 o'clock. Your left knifehand pushes forward and your right hand moves up to protect your head, right palm faces out and your right thumb points down. There is a slight shift forward but don't bend forward at the waist, keep your back upright.

Fan Through Back (front view)   Fan Through Back (side view)

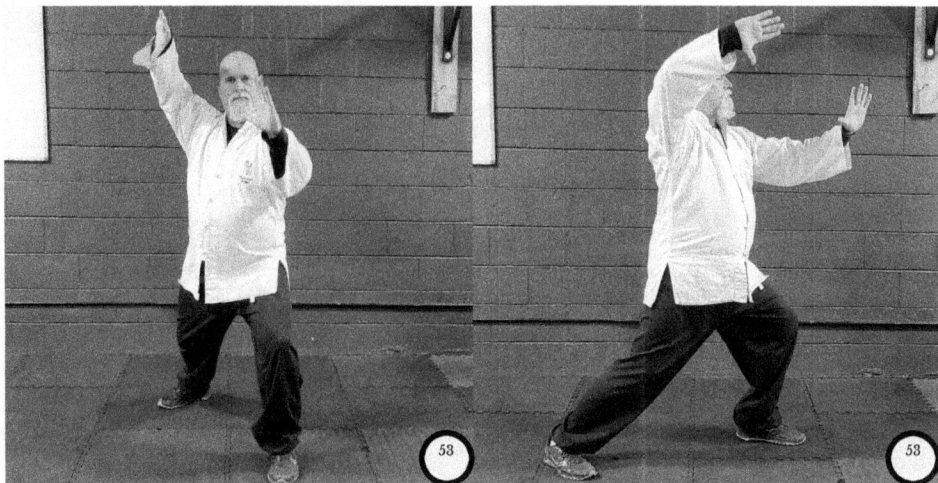

Step Up, Deflect, Parry, and Punch. *54.* Shift your weight to the right, both hands moving to the right at the same time. *55.* Shifting your weight to your left foot, move your left hand to the level of your left shoulder, palm down. Your right hand moves to your left hip in a fist. *56.* Pick up your right foot and place it back down in a twist stance. *57.* Rotate your right foot to the right on your right heel, striking with the back of your right fist as you do so.

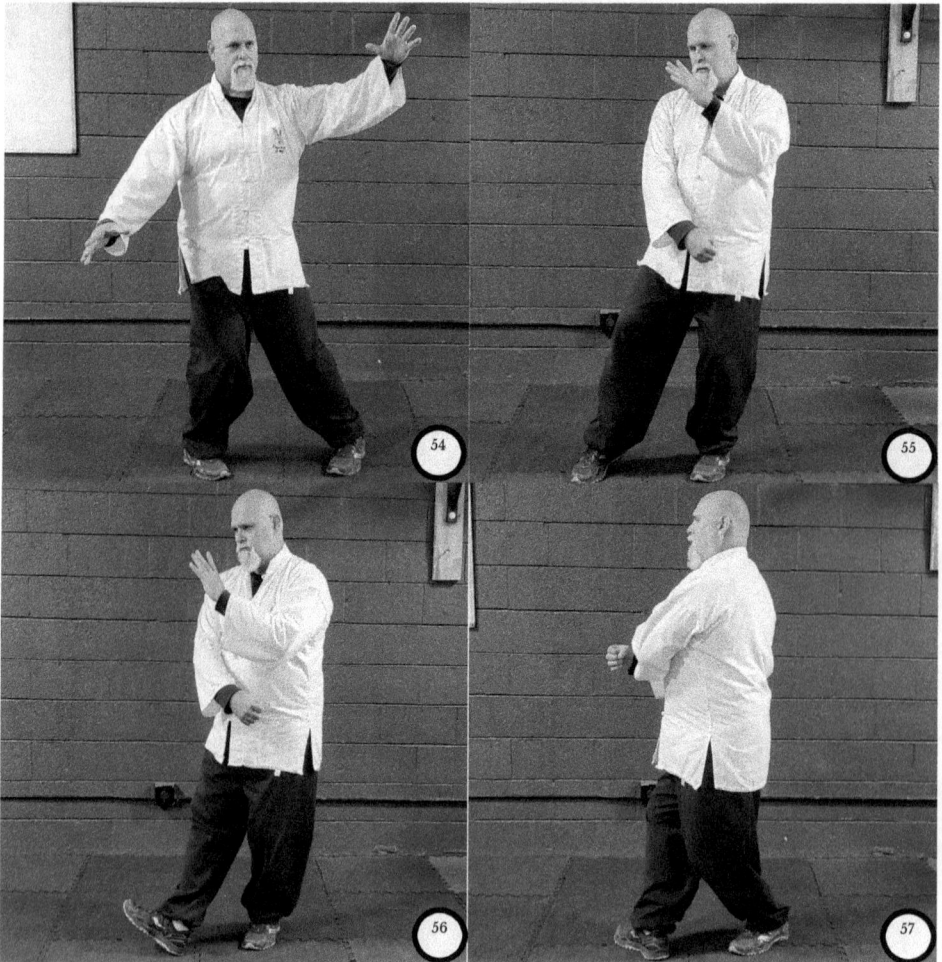

58. Push your left knifehand chop forward. **59**. Step forward towards 9 o'clock with your left foot into a 60/40 stance, right vertical fist punches forward, left hand is palm in at the level of your right elbow. **60**. Bring your left hand to the outside of your right arm (**Picture 60** shows your hand placement from the other side). Left hand scrapes forward down your right arm.

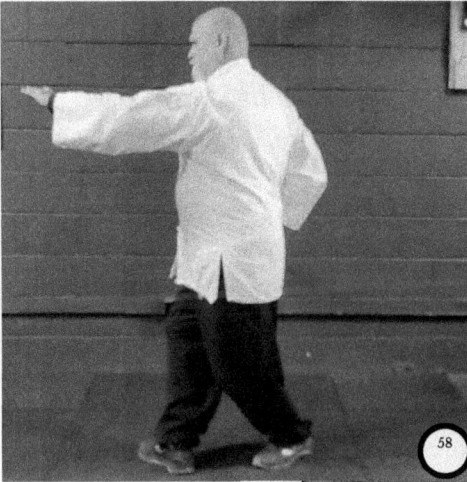

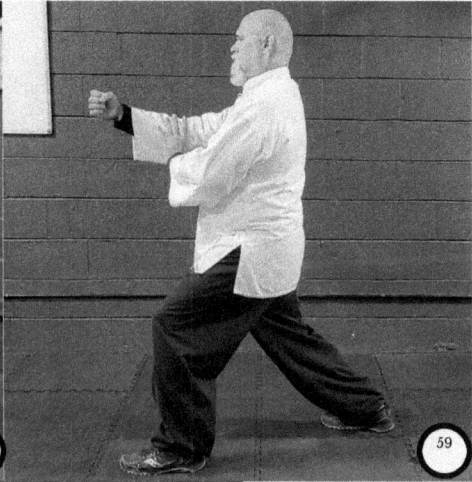

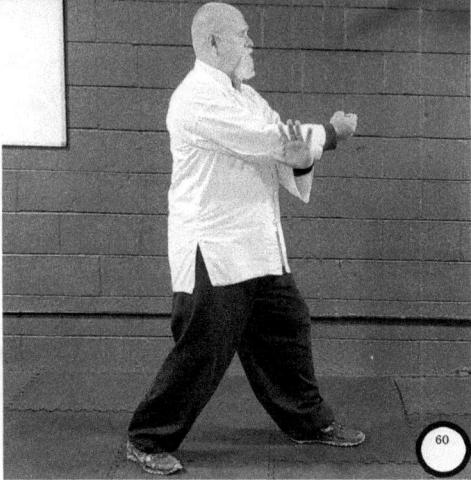

Apparent Withdrawal. 61. Shift your weight back over your right leg and bring both of your hands backwards and down to the level of your *tan tien*. Fingers point down. **62.** Shift your weight forward over your left leg. Two-hand push forward to 9 o'clock with both hands. Palms face out, fingers pointing up. Keep your elbows down.

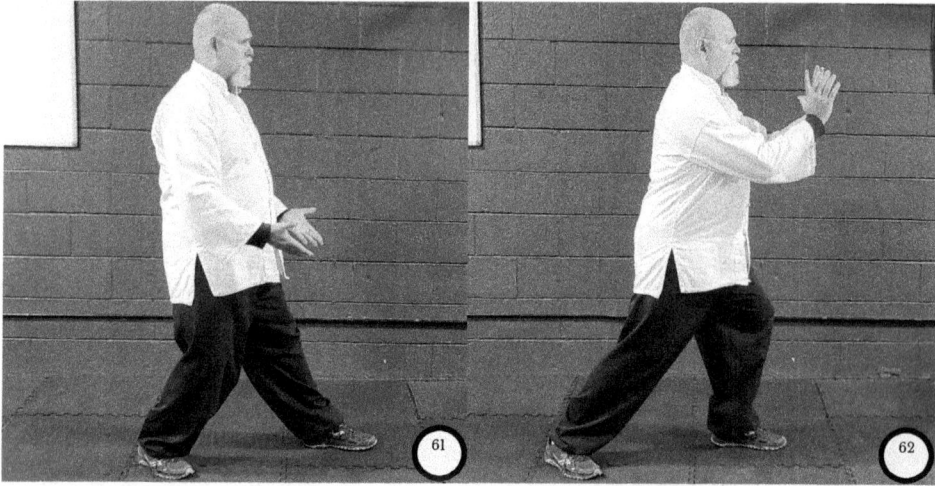

Cross Hands. 63. Shift your weight back onto the right foot. Turn your left foot to the right on your heel turning your body to face 12 o'clock, bring hands above head crossing at the wrists.

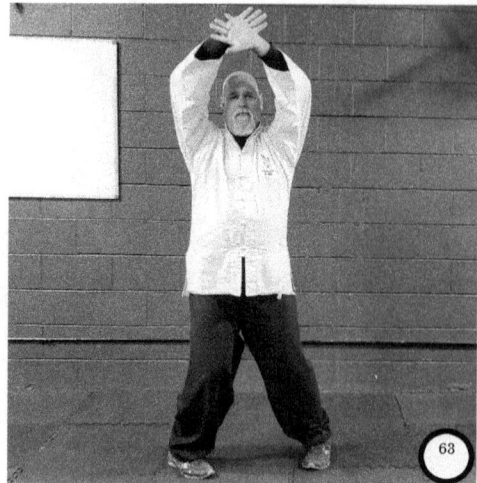

End Tai Chi. Circle both hands out, palms face out, simultaneously bringing your left foot into your right foot. **64**. Your hands finish their motion in front of your *tan tien*. **65**. Then your hands settle at your sides, arms extended down, palms face into the thighs, straight but not locked at the elbows, ending at the position of attention.

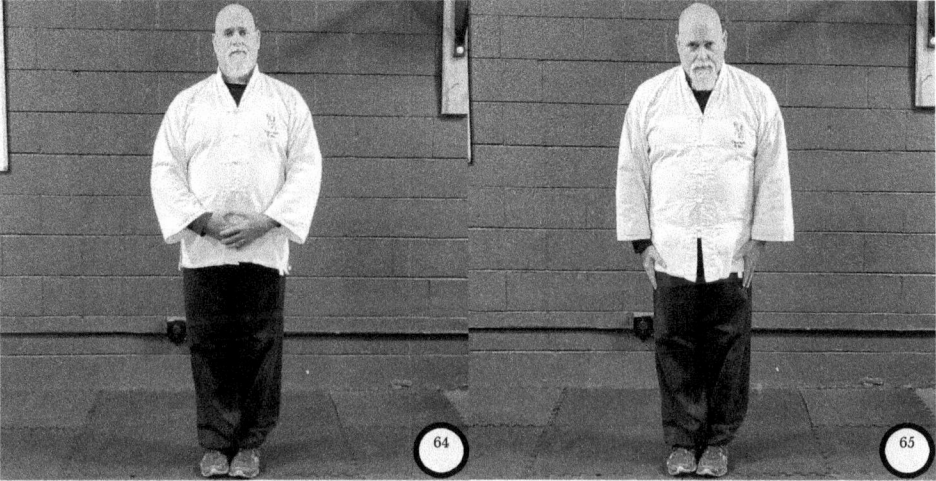

Description of Select Static Postures from the Simplified 24-Move Form

This is an overview of some of the postures found in the empty hand form. Note that there are some differences between the Simplified Form and the Traditional Form. Reference the author's other materials for a more detailed description of the forms. Lead hand and lead foot refer to the hand or foot that is closest to your opponent. The intention of including these descriptions is to assist the student in their practice while learning the form. Understanding the endpoint of each of the following will help you understand the transitions into and out of them.

Attention. Feet together, weight is 50/50. Hands are at sides with your palms resting lightly on your thighs. Head is held erect. Drop the tension in your shoulders. Clear your mind and regulate your breathing—in and out through the nose.

Parting the Wild Horses Mane. Adopt a 60/40 stance. Your lead hand is held at eye level, elbow is bent, palm faces inward. Your back hand is held one fist's distance in front of your hip flexor, fingers pointing forward. Sit both wrists. Keep your torso upright and neutral, do not bend forward at the waist.

White Stork Spreads Wings. Cat stance. Lead hand is held above the level of your head, forearm mostly horizontal but soft with your elbow down. Your back hand is to the side and in the same plane as your lead hand, palm faces down, sit wrist, fingers extend forward.

Brush Knee and Twist Step. Adopt a 60/40 stance. Your lead hand is just to the outside of the knee of your lead leg, fingers facing forwards, palm down, sit the wrist. Your back hand is pushing forward, fingers pointing up, palm faces out, sit the wrist. Both elbows are soft and bent.

Play the Peipa. Adopt a cat stance. Lead hand is open, fingers pointing up, palm is turning in. Your back hand is open, fingers pointing up and palm faces in. Your back hand is at the level of your lead elbow. There should be approximately two fists distance between your palms in front of your midline. Your lead toes are pointing up. Hips and head face forward.

Step Back and Repulse Monkey. Adopt a 60/40 stance (back). Lead hand is held forward, palm out, fingers up, elbow soft. Your back hand is held one fist's distance in front of your *tan tien*, palm up, fingers forward.

Grasp Sparrow's Tail. This has four distinct parts—the description that follows refers to the first one. Adopt a 60/40 stance. Lead hand is at eye level, palm faces in, elbow is soft. Your back hand is at the level of your lead elbow, palm faces in.

Single Whip. Adopt a 60/40 stance. Your lead hand is held at the level of your shoulder, palm faces out, fingers up, sit the wrist. Your back hand is held 90 degrees to the side in a crane beak. The bottoms of the fingers of your crane beak are held at the level of the top of your shoulder. Hips are held 45 degrees off line, but your head faces to the front.

Wave Hands Like Clouds. Small horse stance. One hand is held at the level of your *tan tien*, palm faces in. The other hand is at the level of your eyes palm faces out. Hips are forward. Both knees are slightly bent.

High Pat on Horse. Cat stance, lead toes down. Your lead hand is held in front of your *tan tien*, palm up. Your back hand is head level, palm faces forward, fingers point up. Hips face forward. Both of your hands are in the same plane.

Kick Right. Crane stance. The knee of your lead leg is above the level of your waist. Hips face 45 degrees off the direction you are kicking. Both palms push out.

Creep Low Like Snake. Back knee is bent and back hand is off to the side in a crane break. Lead leg is straight but not locked, and your lead hand generally follows the direction your lead leg is pointing, palm out.

Golden Cock Stands on One Leg. Crane stance. The knee of your lead leg is above the level of your waist. Palms of both hands face inward. Your lead hand is at head level, the palm of your back hand faces the elbow of your lead hand.

Fair Lady Works the Shuttle. Adopt a 60/40 stance. Both palms face out. Your back hand is at stomach level and your lead hand is at head level. Both hands are in the same vertical plane and pushing to the side, fingers extend forward.

Fan Through Back. 60/40 stance. The side of your lead hand pushes forward with your fingers up. Your back hand is up at head level, palm faces out.

Step Up, Deflect, Parry, and Punch. Twist stance. Your back hand is chambered at your hip, palm up but in a fist. Your lead hand is forward, palm down.

Training Transitions

Once the student understands the basics of stances and movement, how to relax, root, and breathe, and can adopt the static postures from the forms, it can be very helpful to go through the transitions from one posture to the next. Transitions are mediated through turning, stepping, and moving the hips.

Although each transitional step between parts of the form is unique, they also follow the same principles as every other piece of tai chi skill development. To practice one part of tai chi is to practice all parts of tai chi.

Some examples of transitions from the Simplified Form to practice with points to pay attention to include:

- Commence Tai Chi to Hold Right Ball. Small horse stance. Turning 90 degrees. Pushing into the ground from a static position to generate force to turn. Coordinating hip and arm movements. Turning waist to move arms.

- Hold Right Ball to Parting the Wild Horses Mane. Stepping forward into 60/40 stance. Chambering. Executing technique from chambered position.

- Parting the Wild Horses Mane to White Stork Spreads Wings. Half step forward. Shifting from 60/40 stance to cat stance.

- Play the Peipa to Step Back and Repulse Monkey. Backwards step shifting to 60/40 stance.

Three Outcomes of Technique

Although beyond the scope of this book, the student should be aware that each technique in tai chi can end in one of three outcomes, determined by the student in the moment.

These three are joint locks (*qin na*), throws or takedowns (*shuai jiao*), and body cavity strikes (*dim mak*).

Joint locks are the manipulations of articulating body parts to damage a joint or use pain compliance to control your opponent. Throws and takedowns are a wide variety of reaps, sweeps, trips, and other off-balancing techniques to bring your opponent to the ground. Body cavity strikes are carefully targeted kinetic blows using your hands or feet to sensitive or vital spots on your opponent's anatomy or acupressure points.

Push Hands (tui shou)

Push hands is arguably the most important training aid in tai chi. It is primarily an exercise requiring a partner, although some limited solo training exists. The value of this exercise comes from allowing a partner to expose weaknesses in your understanding of tai chi principles. The objective of push hands is to recognize and control your partner's intent. It is the only objective way to evaluate your understanding and skill in tai chi. There are many variations and many patterns. It is easy to practice push hands incorrectly and learn the wrong lessons. Push hands is more fully explored through the author's other written materials.

Push hands components:

- Static push hands
    - One hand
    - Two hands
- Dynamic push hands
- Push hands drills

Push hands components

- Physical skill development includes learning how to root, sensitivity training, adhere/stick, power manifestation, silk reeling, breath, *jing* applications etc.

- Energetic skill development includes learning to generate and circulate *qi*, *qi* coiling, sensing and responding to your partner's intention, etc.

Push hands drill.

1. Student One and Student Two face each other in mirrored 60/40 stances. Right hands are crossed, palms facing in, at the wrists. Each partner has their left hand on the other's elbow. **2.** Student Two pushes forward into Student One's right arm. The push comes from Student Two's back leg, not his arms. The arms are a conduit for the force not the generator of the force.

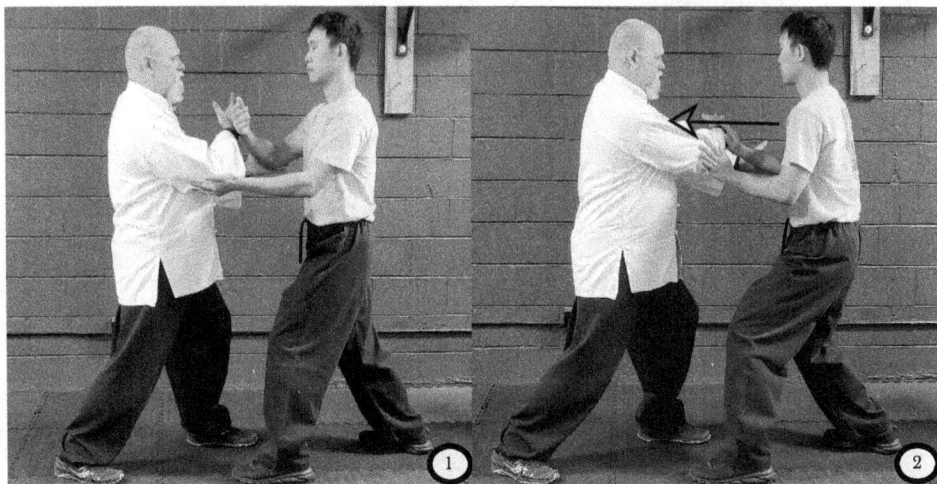

3. Student One lets the force from the push move him back a little onto his back leg. Never let the top of your head move past your heels as this creates an unacceptable condition of instability. **4**. As he settles into his back foot, Student One allows his hips to turn to the right. This gently guides Student Two's energy to the side. As Student Two's force extends forward, Student One pushes Student Two's right arm with his left hand.

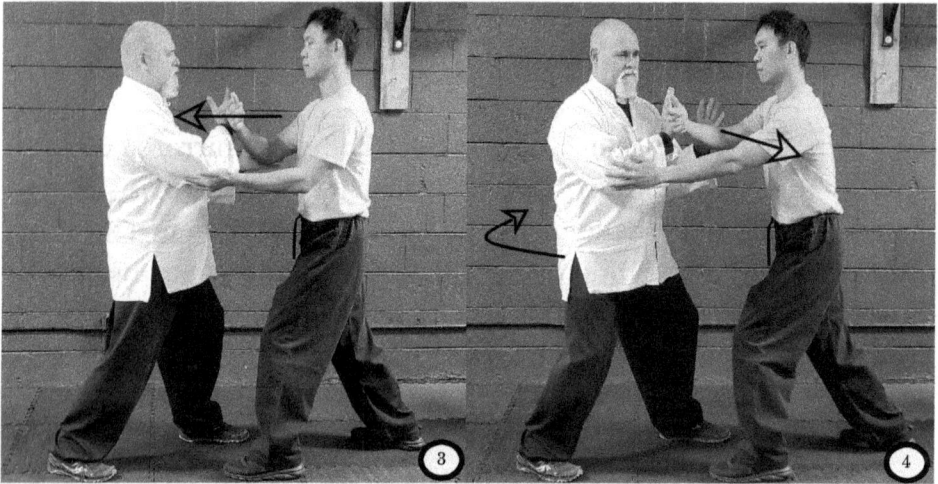

5-6. Student One is now in position to push back into Student Two. He adjusts his hands onto Student Two's right forearm and pushes forward.

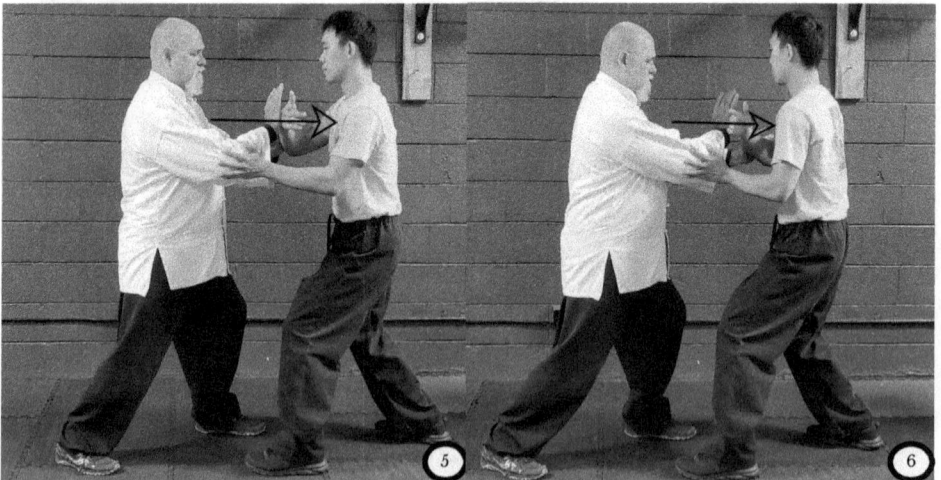

7-8. <u>Student One's</u> attack has finished, <u>Student Two</u> deflects his energy to the side and repositions his hands for his attack. Continue the exchange from the beginning.

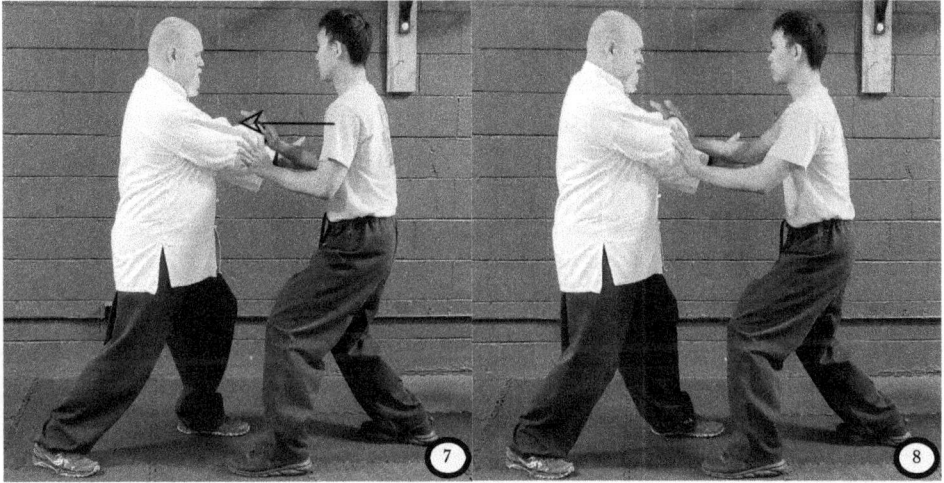

This back-and-forth circular motion continues. In the beginning this drill is done cooperatively—slowly and without too much aggressive power. With more experience, students can increase the tempo. Ultimately the goal is to learn how to relax and redirect unwanted energy coming into your body.

The final stages of push hands incorporates movement, joint locks, and takedowns. This training is reserved for the most advanced students.

The Forms and Their Learning Objectives

Below are the main forms taught at our school, both tai chi forms (empty hand and weapons) and relevant qi gong sets. Included in this list are the learning objectives or purpose of each form. The list of learning objectives is not exhaustive, and there are many ways of modifying your practice to produce different results. Moreover, all of the forms could be simply considered gentle exercise or stretching used to promote health, balance, and fitness. Most of the time spent practicing and learning tai chi is done through the following forms. Descriptions of the forms and their applications can be found in the author's other written materials.

- **Empty hand forms** (Simplified 24-move and Traditional Forms). All of the empty hand forms teach relaxation, sitting the wrist, rooting, and controlling momentum. They introduce what is often referred to as the 13 Postures, or ways of applying technique and movement. With appropriate practice and training, additional skills can be acquired.

    - **Empty hand forms (with proper breath)**. Breath and body integration.

    - **Empty hand forms (with *qi* circulation)**. This is perhaps the pinnacle of tai chi training. Breath, body, and *qi* come together while practicing. The first plateau is the circulate *qi* through the *Ren* and the *Du* channels. The most advanced application is to circulate *qi* through all 12 acupuncture channels.

    - **Empty hand forms (with *jing*/application)**. Pursuit of this skill is an important part of tai chi training, and is limited to more advanced students. Each move in the form can be thought of as an idea that is contextualized in the moment by the practitioner.

- **Empty hand forms (with** *jing*/**application).** In terms of tai chi as a martial art, different energies and outcomes are spontaneously manifested to meet the actions of your opponent in context of the environment. The three potential outcomes are 1. a throw or takedown, **2.** a body cavity strike, or **3.** a joint lock.

- **Minor Universal Qi Gong.** *Qi* cultivation and circulation of *qi* in the *ren* and *du* channels. This can be done as a stand-alone practice, or it can be done while practicing one of the tai chi forms.

- **Major Universal Qi Gong.** Qi cultivation and circulation in the 12 acupuncture channels. This can be done as a stand-alone practice, or it can be done while practicing one of the tai chi forms.

- **Qi Coiling Gong.** Practiced to put *qi* into the bones and to teach the student how to coil *qi.*

- **Tai Chi Qi Gong.** A modern 18-move external qi gong based on the movements of the tai chi forms performed to strengthen the body. Created in the 20th century by a doctor in China who wanted his chronically ill and hospitalized patients to have an exercise that they could do that would benefit their *qi* and speed their recovery.

- **Weapons Forms.** Tai chi weapons forms are rarely practiced for combat. Instead, they provide additional opportunities to challenge the student, teach specific skills, and introduce new concepts. They are generally introduced after the student has achieved proficiency in one of the empty-hand forms.

- **Spear.** The spear used in tai chi is often made of bamboo or waxwood. These materials are light, strong. and flexible. The tai chi spear is also quite long, anywhere from 8 feet to 12 feet in length. The softer wood and great length give the tai chi spear some of the characteristics of a whip. The spear teaches speed, nimbleness, sticking, coiling, agility, circular flow, connection and movement through the *tan tien*, and *fa jing*.

- **Sword.** The tai chi sword is an elegant two-bladed weapon used primarily for stabbing with the sharpened tip. It is sometimes referred to as the "Scholar's sword" because of the long, arduous amount of time it takes to develop skill in. It teaches the student how to extend their *qi*, gracefulness, softness, balance, posture, flow, and lightness. It is the "*yin*" of the two swords found in tai chi.

- **Saber.** Originally a cavalry weapon, it has been co-opted into tai chi. It is the "*yang*" of the two swords found in tai chi. It is a "hand and a half" weapon meaning that although most of the techniques are performed with one hand, it has a longer hilt than the sword allowing some strikes to be executed with two hands. It teaches heaviness, power, root, and concentration.

- **Fan**. A metal folding fan attached to, and held together with delicate sheets of silk. It is used both to strike vital points on the body and slash with the sharpened tips of the metal tines. The fan teaches accuracy, kinetic energy transfer, and *fa jing*.

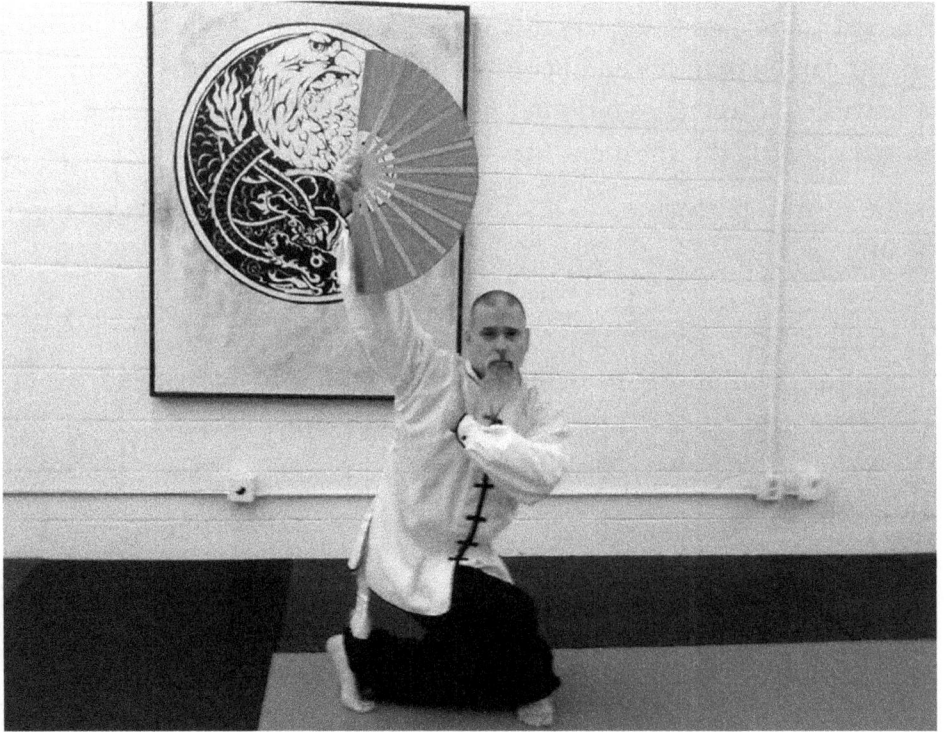

Tai Chi Fan

The Five Elements Form

The Five Elements form is a breathing and internal cultivation movement set. This form originates in a martial art called Chun Kuo Kung Fu and is not a traditional tai chi form. It is included here because it is an excellent supplemental form to your tai chi training. Students should practice rooting and *tan tien* breathing while performing. Additionally, the form allows the student to hone their body structure and alignment while learning about how the five elements can be manifested in combat. While practicing this form pay attention to directing your energies as indicated by the element and understanding the momentum.

The form is performed to the four cardinal directions. Start facing South.

- **Salutation. 1.** Start facing to 12 o'clock at attention with your palms on your thighs. Bring the back of your hands to the front of your thighs. **2.** Move your arms out to either side. Inhale through the nose as your arms go up.

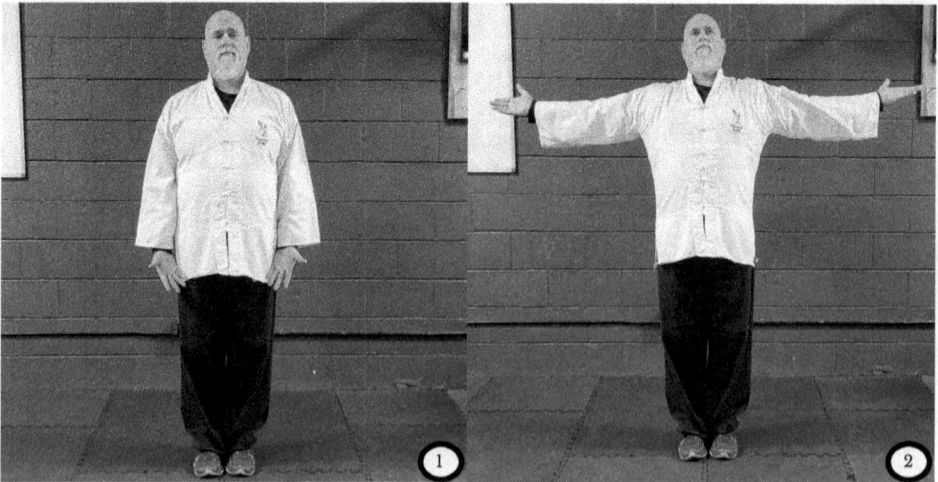

- **Salutation. 3**. Continue until your arms are over your head. **4**. Palms turn down and your hands move downward until the fingers of both hands point towards each other at chest level. Exhale as you push down. **5**. Push hands down to the level of your *tan tien*, palms facing down, fingers still facing each other.

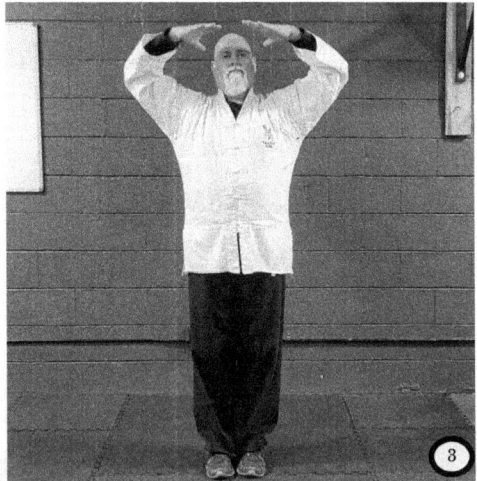

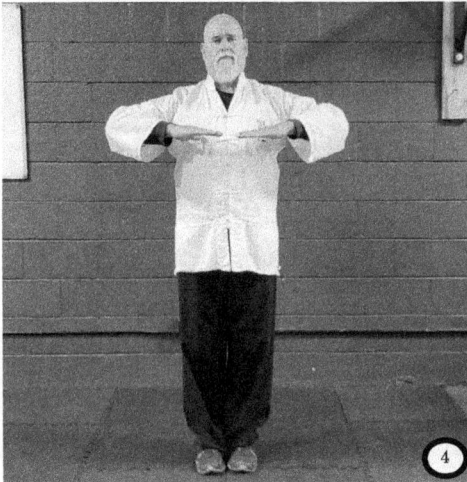

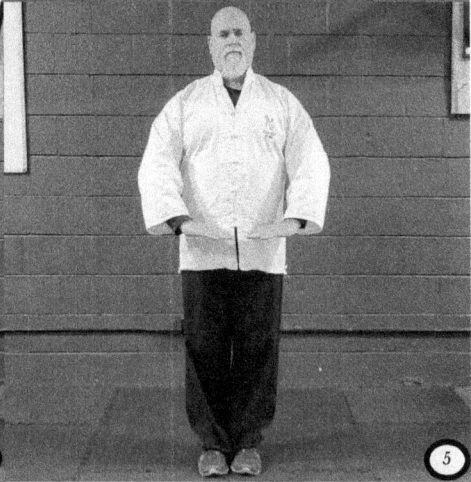

- **Fire. 6**. Move into a cat stance, shifting your weight to your right leg. Step forward with the left foot into a 60/40 stance, both of your hands chamber to the right side.

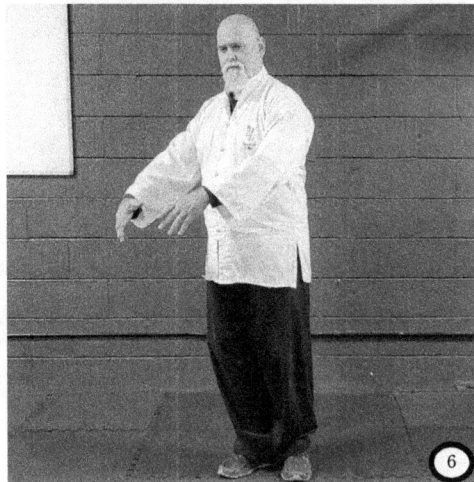

7. Both hands rise to chest level palms face down. **8**. Both hands begin to drop, palms face forward. Step forward leading with the heel of your left foot.

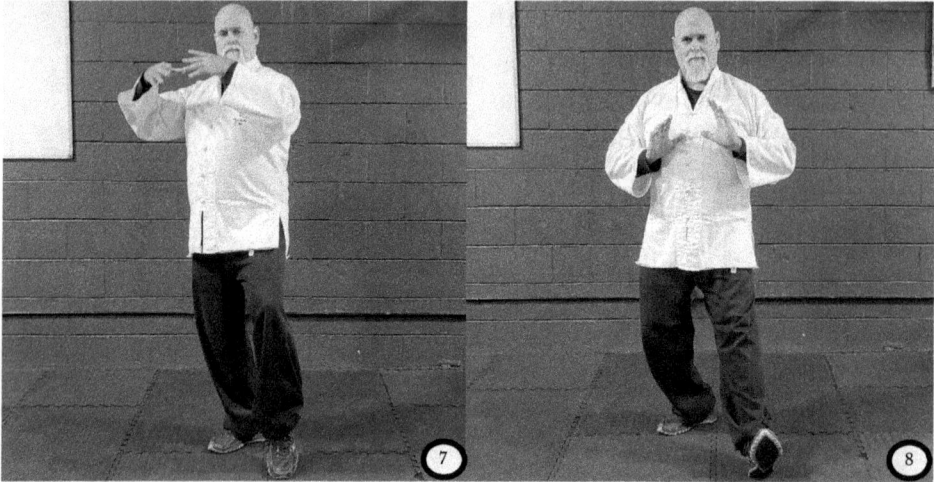

9-10. As you shift your weight forward ending in a 60/40 stance, two-hand push from your *tan tien*. Hands go from low to high ending at chest level. The power of this push comes from your back leg, not your arms. The nature of Fire is to go forward and up. Its strategy is to attack, and its energy corresponds to the Tiger.

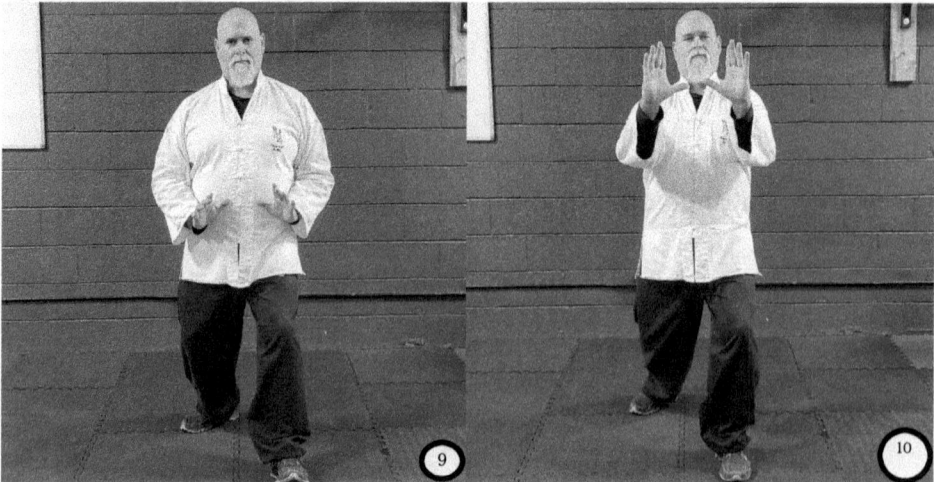

- **Water. 11.** Still facing 12 o'clock, pull back into a cat stance with your left leg forward. Scoop arms backwards, palms facing in towards your chest and push down, dropping your body and your energy down. Sit back slightly but keep your head and your spine in alignment. The nature of Water is to flow, yield, and move backwards. It is the counter to the offensive and linear power of Fire. Its strategy is to be defensive and circular. Its energy corresponds to Crane.

Water (side view)   Water (front view)

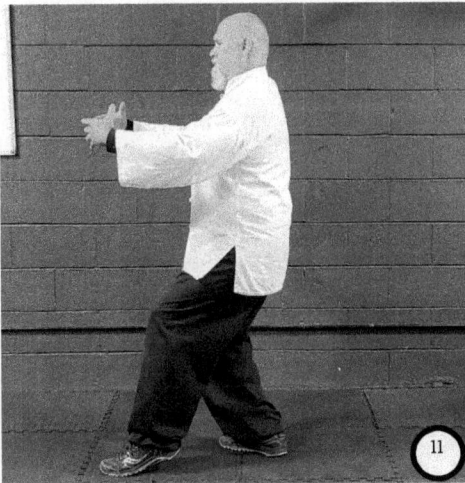

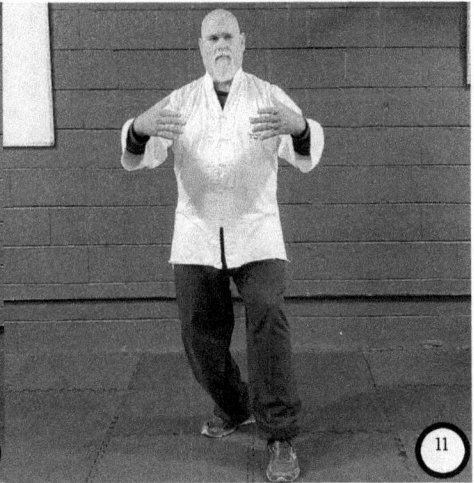

- **Wood.** **12.** Continue facing 12 o'clock. Transition from a cat stance (from the previous move) into a traditional horse stance by stepping your left leg back and to the left. Your hands cross at the wrists. **13-14.** Your hands drop down and begin to circle out and up. **15.** Push hands out to the sides, palms facing out. The nature of Wood is to expand and move outwards. Its strategy is to use angles to surprise its opponent. Its energy corresponds to Leopard.

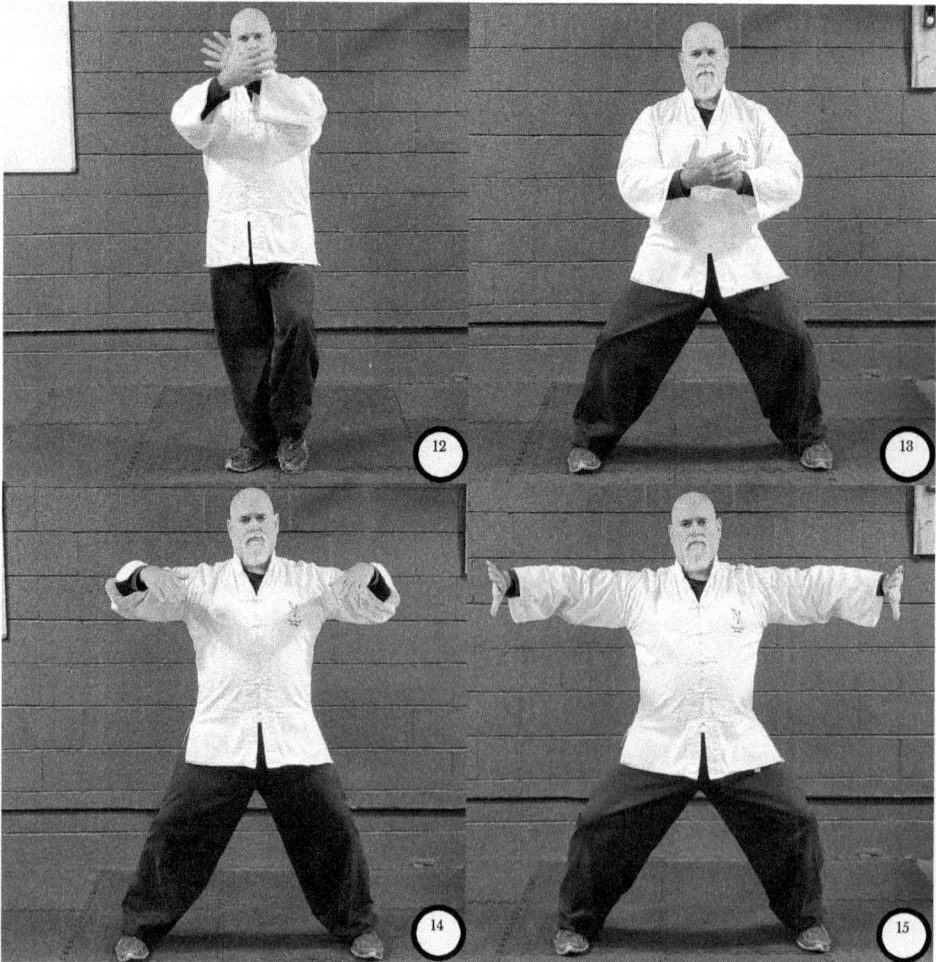

- **Earth. 16.** Move into a tiger-snake twist stance turning to the right. Both hands come in. Turn your left foot in on the heel. **17-18.** Turn your right foot out on the heel. Turn your torso to the right. **19.** Settle into a tiger-snake twist stance facing 9 o'clock. Both hands move into a guard position. The nature of Earth is to be rooted and balanced. Its strategy is to be unyielding while at the same time using its rooted stance to deflect an attack to either side. Its energy corresponds to Dragon.

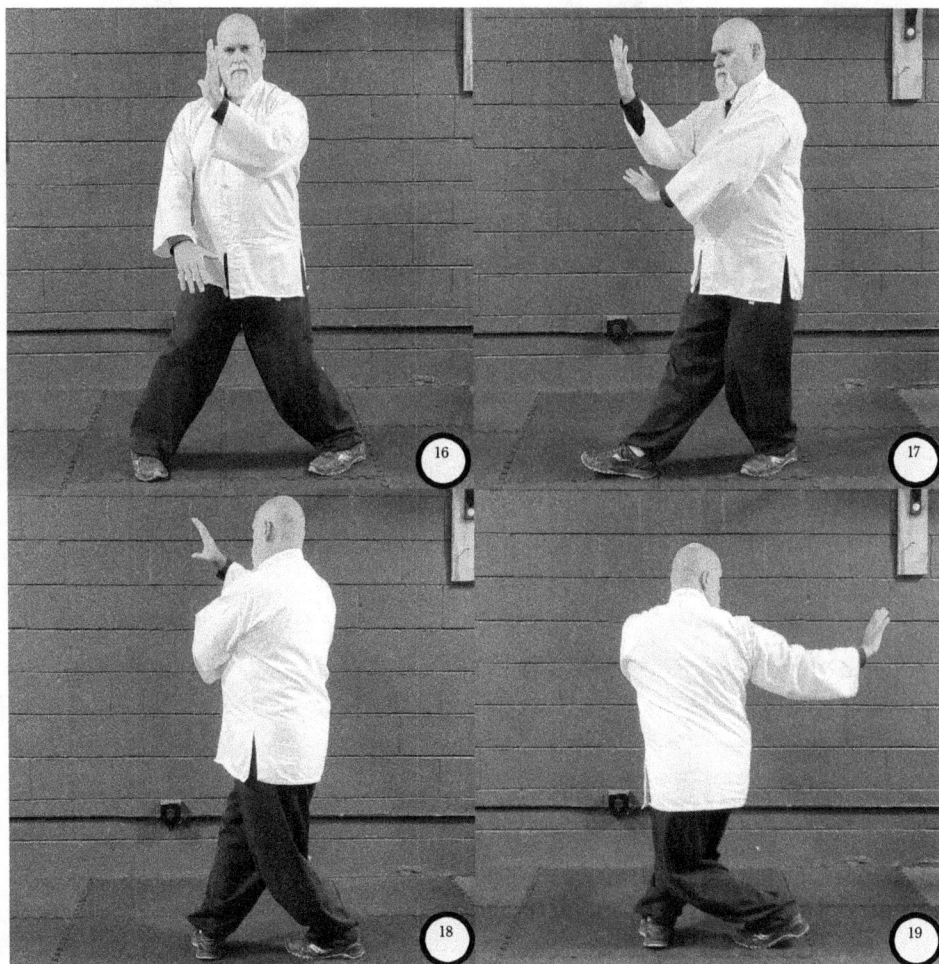

- **Metal. 20.** Move out of the tiger-snake twist stance (from the previous move) by stepping through with left foot into a horse stance. You will end up facing to 3 o'clock. Arms cross at the wrists. **21.** Circle both hands down and out, palms face out.

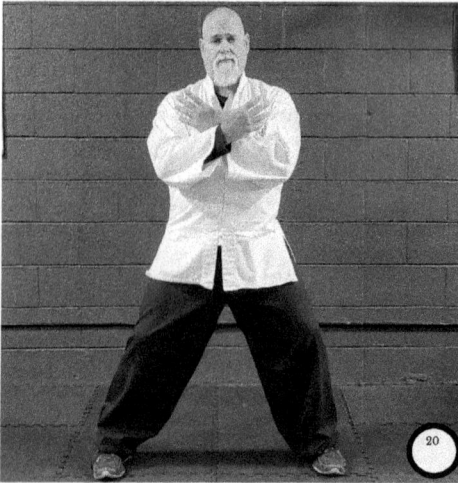

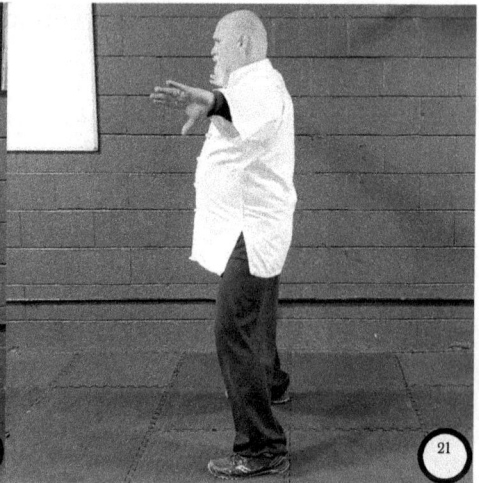

22. Bring both hands together, palms facing each other and touching. The nature of Metal is to consolidate and move inward. Its energy corresponds to Snake.

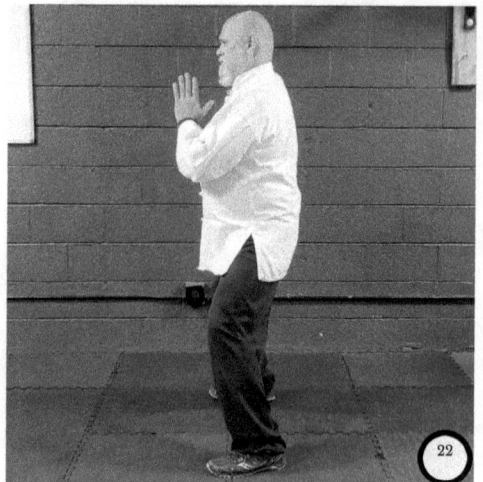

Closing Salutation. 23. End the form facing 12 o'clock at attention, using the same salutation the form began with. Repeat each of the previous steps in the remaining three cardinal directions—West, North, and East.

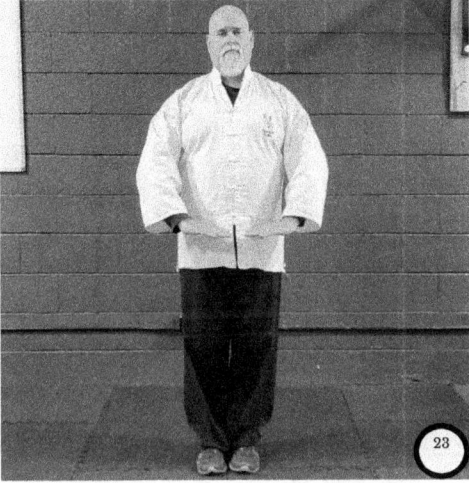

Appendix

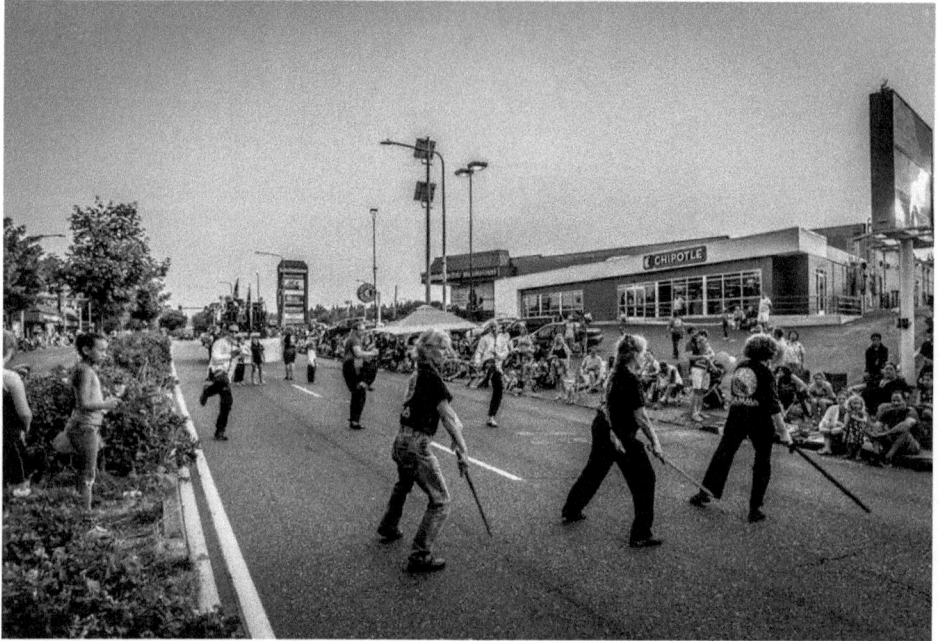

Tai Chi Performance

Seafair Parade, Seattle

2017

Glossary of Chinese Terms

The following transliterated Chinese words appear in this text.

An. Push. One of the Eight Energies.

Bagua (or pakua, pakwa). Refers to the Eight Trigrams. The eight principle energies in tai chi that form the basis of technique and martial application.

Cai. Pluck. One of the Eight Energies.

Dao yin. Longevity exercises.

Dim mak. Refers to the art and science of striking specific vulnerable spots on the body.

Du (channel). One of the Extraordinary Channels. This is the repository of *yang qi* in your body.

Fa jing. Explosive power.

Hun. The spirit of the Liver. This is also your ethereal body, the part of you that lives on after the physical body dies.

Ji. Press. One of the Eight Energies.

Jing (or jin). System of power generation.

Kau. Shoulder stroke. One of the Eight Energies.

Kua (or kwa). The inguinal crease and hip joint.

Li. Muscle strength.

Lie. Split. One of the Eight Energies.

Lu. Rollback. One of the Eight Energies.

Peng. Wardoff. One of the Eight Energies.

P'o. The spirit of the Lung. This is your corporeal body. Returns to the earth upon death.

Qi (or chi). Internal energy or vital force.

Qin na. The study and application of joint locks.

Qi gong (or chi gong). Refers to many different exercises intended to enhance our connection to and understanding of internal energy.

Ren (channel). One of the Extraordinary Channels. This is the repository of *yin qi* in your body.

Shen. Spirit of the Heart. Refers to the collection of psychological, spiritual, and emotional parts of our lives.

Shuai jiao. The study and application of throws and takedowns.

Song. Refers to a body structure that is soft but rooted and structurally sound. Relaxed but structurally sound.

Tan tien (or dan tien). A spot in our abdomen between the kidneys where we store qi.

Taoism (or Daoism). Ancient Chinese spiritual practice concerned with longevity practices and internal alchemy.

Tui shou. Push hands.

Wu ji. The metaphysical state of nothingness that exists before starting the practice of tai chi.

Wu shen. The Five Spirits. Each of the main internal organs is associated with one. Spleen (yi), Kidney (zhi), Lung (p'o), Liver (hun), and Heart (shen).

Yi. Spirit of the Spleen. Your intention.

Yin/yang. Theory about how two related things can be compared and contrasted.

Zang Fu. The twelve organs in TCM. They are the basis for pathology and diagnosis.

Zhi. The spirit of the Kidney. Your willpower.

Zou. Elbow stroke. One of the Eight Energies.

The following classical books are referenced in this text.

I Ching. Classic of Changes. An ancient book, originating in China in antiquity. Introduces a historically important system of divination.

Tao Te Ching. Classic of the Tao. An ancient book that is the fundamental text of Taoism.

Tai Chi for Medical Conditions

When combined with standard treatment, tai chi appears to be helpful for several medical conditions. This is a partial list (9). Examples include:

- *Arthritis.* In a 40-person study at Tufts University, presented in October 2008 at a meeting of the American College of Rheumatology, an hour of tai chi twice a week for 12 weeks reduced pain and improved mood and physical functioning more than standard stretching exercises in people with severe knee osteoarthritis. According to a Korean study published in December 2008 in *Evidence-based Complementary and Alternative Medicine*, eight weeks of tai chi classes followed by eight weeks of home practice significantly improved flexibility and slowed the disease process in patients with ankylosing spondylitis, a painful and debilitating inflammatory form of arthritis that affects the spine.

- *Low bone density.* A review of six controlled studies by Dr. Wayne and other Harvard researchers indicates that tai chi may be a safe and effective way to maintain bone density in postmenopausal women. A controlled study of tai chi in women with osteopenia (diminished bone density not as severe as osteoporosis) is under way at the Osher Research Center and Boston's Beth Israel Deaconess Medical Center.

- *Breast cancer.* Tai chi has shown potential for improving quality of life and functional capacity (the physical ability to carry out normal daily activities, such as work or exercise) in women suffering from breast cancer or the side effects of breast cancer treatment. For example, a 2008 study at the University of Rochester, published in *Medicine and Sport Science*, found that quality of life and functional capacity (including aerobic capacity, muscular strength, and flexibility) improved in women with breast cancer who did 12 weeks of tai chi, while declining in a control group that received only supportive therapy.

- *Heart disease.* A 53-person study at National Taiwan University found that a year of tai chi significantly boosted exercise capacity, lowered blood pressure, and improved levels of cholesterol, triglycerides, insulin, and C-reactive protein in people at high risk for heart disease. The study, which was published in the September 2008 Journal of *Alternative and Complementary Medicine*, found no improvement in a control group that did not practice tai chi.

- *Heart failure.* In a 30-person pilot study at Harvard Medical School, 12 weeks of tai chi improved participants' ability to walk and quality of life. It also reduced blood levels of B-type natriuretic protein, an indicator of heart failure. A 150-patient controlled trial is underway.

- *Hypertension.* In a review of 26 studies in English and Chinese published in *Preventive Cardiology* (Spring 2008), Dr. Yeh reported that in 85% of trials, tai chi lowered blood pressure — with improvements ranging from 3 to 32 mm Hg in systolic pressure and from 2 to 18 mm Hg in diastolic pressure.

- *Parkinson's disease.* A 33-person pilot study from Washington University School of Medicine in St. Louis, published in *Gait and Posture* (October 2008), found that people with mild to moderately severe Parkinson's disease showed improved balance, walking ability, and overall well-being after 20 tai chi sessions.

- *Sleep problems.* In a University of California, Los Angeles study of 112 healthy older adults with moderate sleep complaints, 16 weeks of tai chi improved the quality and duration of sleep significantly more than standard sleep education. The study was published in the July 2008 issue of the journal *Sleep*.

Thoughts about the Practice of Tai Chi from
Dr. Boonchai Apichai

- "Even if you practice tai chi wrong, it's better than if you don't practice at all."

- "Practice tai chi to get it, practice to forget it."

- "Never lock your elbows during tai chi practice."

- "Imagine that there is a string from the sky tied to your head pulling your head up."

- "In tai chi we have to relax."

- "In tai chi the term for bending the wrist is called 'sit'; you 'sit' the wrist. You 'sink' the shoulders and you 'sink' the elbows."

- "We say tai chi is like moving meditation; you're doing the move, but you don't focus on the outside you focus on the inside."

- "People practice the same form forever. One form is enough for a whole lifetime. You can always find mistakes."

- "Tai chi is very good for people of every age."

- "In tai chi you need to empty your mind during practice."

- "Let your muscles learn tai chi, not your brain."

- "Tai chi is always opposite, when your hands are down, your qi is going up."

- "Never lock the joints in tai chi."

- "In tai chi, the waist is the Commander."

- "Tai chi is continuous, keep the hands and feet moving all the time. Muscles are moving all the time; joints are moving all the time"

- "The faster moving hand is the *Yang* hand. Your eyes should be on the *Yang* hand."

- "In tai chi practice there are three levels. The first is to practice the structure, the second is to be able to be empty. The third is to use your mind to lead your movements."

- "Tai chi is that once you finish the move you have to immediately go to the next move."

- "Tai chi brings us back to nature."

The Twelve Acupuncture Channels

The following list details the major acupuncture channels and their associations. These channels connect every molecule in your body. They explain how *qi* is able to move from place to place. Each channel connects to one of the twelve internal *Zang Fu* organs. *Zang Fu* organ theory is the basis of pathology and diagnosis in Traditional Chinese Medicine.

The following outlines the name of the channel, its standard abbreviation, the time the qi is most active in the channel, whether the channel is a *Yin* channel or a *Yang* channel, and the channel's corresponding element.

- **Lung** (LU) 3 am-5 am, *Yin* channel, Metal.
- **Large Intestine** (LI) 5 am-7 am *Yang* channel, Metal.
- **Stomach** (ST) 7 am-9 am *Yang* channel, Earth.
- **Spleen** (SP) 9 am-11 am *Yin* channel, Earth.
- **Heart** (HT) 11 am-1 pm *Yin* channel, Fire.
- **Small Intestine** (SI) 1pm-3 pm *Yang* channel, Fire.
- **Urinary Bladder** (UB) 3 pm-5 pm *Yang* channel, Water.
- **Kidney** (KD) 5 pm–7 pm *Yin* channel, Water.
- **Pericardium** (PC) 7 pm-9 pm *Yin* channel, Fire.
- **San Jiao** (SJ) 9 pm –11 pm *Yang* channel, Fire.
- **Gallbladder** (GB) 11 pm-1 am *Yang* channel, Wood.
- **Liver** (LV) 1 am-3 am *Yin* channel, Wood.

The Organs and their Associated Emotions

An in-depth understanding of Traditional Chinese Medicine is certainly not required for the practice of tai chi. However, some general knowledge of TCM can be helpful in understanding some of the deeper meanings and effects of your practice, and may help improve your overall health.

TCM teaches that our health goals can be better obtained through balance in all things. Too much food, not enough exercise, and even the management of our emotions can negatively affect our health.

Experiencing emotional highs and lows is a normal part of being human and something that we all share. However, our *qi* is influenced by feelings of long-term, excess or inappropriate emotions. For example, holding onto grief can damage the Lung *qi*, letting stress or anger run unfettered can damage the Liver *qi*. The following organs are particularly affected by the associated emotion.

- **Lung**—grief.
- **Spleen**—worry.
- **Heart**—joy.
- **Kidney**—fear.
- **Liver**—anger.

The practice of tai chi can help regulate and move stuck *qi* to help keep our emotions from getting the better of us.

Five Element Correspondences

This table shows the relationships between nature (as expressed through the five elements) and various aspects of your *qi*. Although not directly related to the practice of tai chi, they form an important part of understanding health and wellness as viewed through the lens of Traditional Chinese Medicine.

Element	Fire	Earth	Metal	Water	Wood
Yin Organ	Heart Pericardium	Spleen	Lung	Kidney	Liver
Yang Organ	Small Intestine San Jiao	Stomach	Large Intestine	Urinary Bladder	Gallbladder
Season	Summer	Late Summer	Fall	Winter	Spring
Climate	Heat	Damp	Dry	Cold	Wind
Emotion	Joy	Worry	Grief	Fear	Anger
Sense Organ	Tongue	Mouth	Nose	Ears	Eyes
Taste	Bitter	Sweet	Pungent	Salty	Sour
Sound	Laughing	Singing	Crying	Groaning	Shouting
Smell	Scorched	Fragrant	Rotten	Putrid	Rancid
Tissue	Blood Vessels	Muscles	Skin	Bones	Tendons

Tai Chi Competencies

Theory

- Explain what tai chi is and give three reasons why one should learn it.
- State your tai chi lineage and explain why it is important to know.
- Explain the purpose of muscle tensing.
- Demonstrate how to perform five different muscle tensing exercises.
- Describe three other relaxation techniques.
- List five ways you can practice tai chi outside of class.
- List five benefits from practicing tai chi.
- Describe the cosmology of tai chi.
- Name all ten components of tai chi.
- Demonstrate the tai chi salutation and explain its symbology.
- Define *qi* and describe where it comes from and how we can get more.
- Describe the consequences for having a *qi* imbalance.
- Describe symptoms related to stagnant *qi.*
- Describe symptoms related to deficient *qi.*
- Explain yin/yang theory.
- List the five laws of yin/yang theory and explain each.
- Name each part of the yin/yang symbol with its corresponding law.
- Broadly describe how *yin* and *yang* manifest during tai chi practice.
- Define the *tan tien* and give its location.

- List the two functions of the *tan tien*.

- Explain five elements theory.

- Name each of the five elements.

- Ascribe a quality of movement to each of the five elements.

- Describe the Three Taoist Treasures and how tai chi help us cultivate them.

- List three important acupressure points, include their location on the body and what they are used for.

- Define *jing*, and contrast it to *li*.

- List the four categories of *jing* development.

- Explain how we integrate breathing into our tai chi practice and explain its importance.

- Describe natural breathing.

- Describe how to breathe in accordance with the rules of *yin* and *yang*.

- Describe opening, absorbing, yielding, breaking, opening, and expanding as they apply to the Eight Energies.

- Demonstrate one example of each of the following bagua or Eight Energies – elbow stroke, pluck, press, push, rollback, shoulder stroke, split, wardoff.

- Explain the meaning and symbolism of the salutation.

Warm-Ups, Stretches, and Exercises

- Describe how rotations are different than stretches.

- Demonstrate each of the following rotations – neck, arm and shoulder, wrist, hips, knees, and ankles.

- Describe the benefits to performing rotations.

- Demonstrate 10 different stretches.

- Demonstrate 10 warm-up exercises.

Training and Development

- Demonstrate the following static postures—Parting the Wild Horses Mane, White Stork Spreads Wings, Brush Knee and Twist Step, Play the Peipa, Wardoff, Press, Push, Single Whip, High Pat on Horse, Snake Creeps Low, Golden Cock Stands on One Leg, Push Needle to Sea Bottom, Fan Through Back.

Basics

- Demonstrate each of the following stances and hold each for 30 seconds on both sides (if applicable): attention, traditional horse stance, small horse stance, cat stance, crane stance, 60/40 stance, snake creeps low.

- Define root.

- Demonstrate root against a partner's push in both a 60/40 stance and a horse stance.

- Demonstrate each of the following hand forms: 2nd MCP, back fist, Buddha palm, crane beak, knife hand chop, knife hand thrust, palm heel, ridge hand, sword hand, tai chi fist.

- Demonstrate how each of the above hand forms is used.

- Demonstrate the following kicks: crescent kick, heel kick, toe kick.

- Demonstrate "holding a ball".

- Demonstrate "sitting the wrist".

- Demonstrate opening and closing the *kua*.

- Demonstrate each of the following steps: tai chi step, half step, back step, side step.

- Demonstrate how to turn 180-degrees to change direction of movement.

- Demonstrate tai chi walking both forward, backwards, and to the side.

- Demonstrate the difference between the step in the Simplified Form and the step in the Traditional Form.

- Demonstrate tai chi walking with the following hand movements – Parting the Wild Horses Mane, Brush Knee and Twist Step, Step Back and Repulse Monkey, Wave Hands Like Clouds.

- Demonstrate one-hand static push hands with a partner.

- Demonstrate two-hand static push hands with a partner.

- List the three possible outcomes of technique.

- Demonstrate one of each—joint lock, body cavity strike, and throw.

Training and Development

- Demonstrate the following transitional moves—Commence Tai Chi to Hold Right Ball, Hold Left Ball to Parting the Wild Horses Mane, White Stork Spreads Wings to Brush Knee and Twist Step, Step Back and Repulse Monkey to Grasp Sparrow's Tail, Grasp Sparrow's Tail (left) to Grasp Sparrow's Tail (right), Single Whip to Wave Hands Like Clouds, High Pat on Horse to Kick Right, Snake Creeps Low to Golden Cock Stands on One Leg.

- Describe the process of generating and circulating *qi.*

- Demonstrate five tai chi physical training drills.

- Demonstrate two tai chi energetic training drills.

The Forms

- Demonstrate the 24-Move Simplified Form.

- Demonstrate the 108-Move Traditional Form.

- Demonstrate the Tai Chi Qi Gong Set.

- Demonstrate the Qi Coiling Gong.

- Demonstrate the Five Elements Form.

- Demonstrate the following weapons forms:

  - Spear Form

  - 32-Sword Form

  - 67-Sword Form

  - Saber Form

  - Fan Form

Academic Competencies

- Define *wu ji*.
- Describe *ding*.
- Describe substantial vs. unsubstantial.
- Describe what it means to be double weighted.
- Explain the purpose behind touching the tongue to the roof of the mouth.
- List the "five spirits", what each translates to, their associated *zang fu* organ, and what aspect of our life each is connected with.
- Describe how *shen* is specifically used in tai chi.
- Describe how *yi* is specifically used in tai chi.
- Give an example of a yin/yang pairing.
- Describe what it means to cultivate *qi*.
- Describe the *qi* sensation and how one might go about inducing it.
- Explain the importance of relaxation to the practice of tai chi.
- List six benefits that one might receive from relaxation.
- List the 13 Postures.
- Explain the importance of the 13 Postures.
- Describe the difference between the Five Elements and the *bagua* as they pertain to the 13 Postures.
- Describe each of the five elements in terms of their martial applications, and give an example of each found in a technique from the empty hand form.

- Describe how rotations help the practice of tai chi.

- Describe how stretching helps the practice of tai chi.

- Define stance.

- Describe how you find the lines of stability and instability in a stance.

- Describe *song*.

- Describe momentum and its relevance to tai chi.

- Describe the path of both the Ren and Du channels, include pertinent anatomical markers.

- List the five traditional weapons found in tai chi.

- Explain what is meant by "chambering".

- Describe the learning objectives of the following forms – Traditional Form, Minor Universal Qi Gong, Major Universal Qi Gong, Qi Coiling Gong, Tai Chi Qi Gong, Spear Form, Sword Forms, Saber Form, Fan Form.

Works Cited

1. Yu-Ning Hu, Yu-Ju Chung, Hui-Kung Yu, Yu-Chi Chen, Chien-Tsung Tsai, Gwo-Chi Hu. "Effect of Tai Chi Exercise on Fall Prevention in Older Adults: Systematic Review and Meta-analysis of Randomized Controlled Trials". Science Direct. https://www.sciencedirect.com/science/article/pii/S1873959816300746

2. Klaudia J. Ćwiękała-Lewis MSN, BSN, RN, APHN-BC, Matthew Gallek PhD, RN, Ruth E. Taylor-Piliae PhD, RN, FAHA. "The effects of Tai Chi on physical function and well-being among persons with Parkinson's Disease: A systematic review". Science Direct. https://www.sciencedirect.com/science/article/abs/pii/S1360859216300997

3. Ching Lan, Ssu-Yuan Chen, Jin-Shin Lai, and Alice May-Kuen Wong. "Tai Chi Chuan in Medicine and Health Promotion". Hindawi. https://www.hindawi.com/journals/ecam/2013/502131/

4. Yannan Chen, PhD; Jiawei Qin, PhD; Liyuan Tao, MD, PhD. "Effects of Tai Chi Chuan on Cognitive Function in Adults 60 Years or Older With Type 2 Diabetes and Mild Cognitive Impairment in China A Randomized Clinical Trial" JAMA Network. https://jamanetwork.com/journals/jamanetworkopen/fullarticle/2803247#:~:text=Another%20study12%20showed%20that,adults%20with%20T2D%20and%20MCI

5. "Tai chi: Promising for COPD". Harvard Health Publishing. https://www.health.harvard.edu/diseases-and-conditions/tai-chi-promising-for-copd

6. Gowri Raman, MD MS, Yuan Zhang, PhD, RN, Vincent J Minichiello, MD, Carolyn M. D'Ambrosio, MD, MS, and Chenchen Wang, MD, MSc. "Tai Chi Improves Sleep Quality in Healthy Adults and Patients with Chronic Conditions: A Systematic Review and Meta-analysis." National Library of Medicine. https://www.ncbi.nlm.nih.gov/pmc/articles/PMC5570448/

7. "Tai Chi What You Need to Know". National Institute for Complimentary and Integrative Health. https://www.nccih.nih.gov/health/tai-chi-what-you-need-to-know

8. "Benefits of Physical Activity". Centers for Disease Control and Prevention. https://www.cdc.gov/physicalactivity/basics/pa-health/. Sep 2023.

9. "The Health Benefits of Tai Chi". Harvard Medical School. May 2009, http://www.health.harvard.edu/newsletters/Harvard_Womens_Health_Watch/2009/May/The-health-benefits-of-tai-chi.

About the Author

Daniel Cashman is the owner of Seattle Asian Medicine and Martial Arts (SAMMA) and the Head Instructor of Chun Kuo Kung Fu. Graduating from Bastyr University in 2008 with a master's degree in Acupuncture and Oriental Medicine, Daniel is a nationally board-certified acupuncturist and is a licensed Acupuncture and East Asian Medicine Practitioner (AEMP) in the State of Washington. He maintains a full time Traditional Chinese Medicine clinic in Seattle which doubles as the home of Chun Kuo Kung Fu and Tai Chi.

Daniel's training in the martial arts began in 1987 at TRACO Kenpo's Glendale Dojo under Mr. Jeff Coronado. He began studying Chun Kuo Kung Fu with the Family of Many Dragons in 1988 under the tutelage of Sifu Robert Brown. He currently holds a White Sash (Instructor) in Chun Kuo Kung Fu under Sifu Robert Brown. In 2004, Daniel began studying tai chi in earnest, and currently is a student of Dr. Boonchai Apichai in Seattle, WA.

In addition to a lifetime of martial arts training, Daniel has been a professional musician, as well as an Arabic language interpreter. Prior to becoming an acupuncturist, Daniel spent 10 years in the U.S. Army as both an Artillery Forward Observer and an Interrogator.

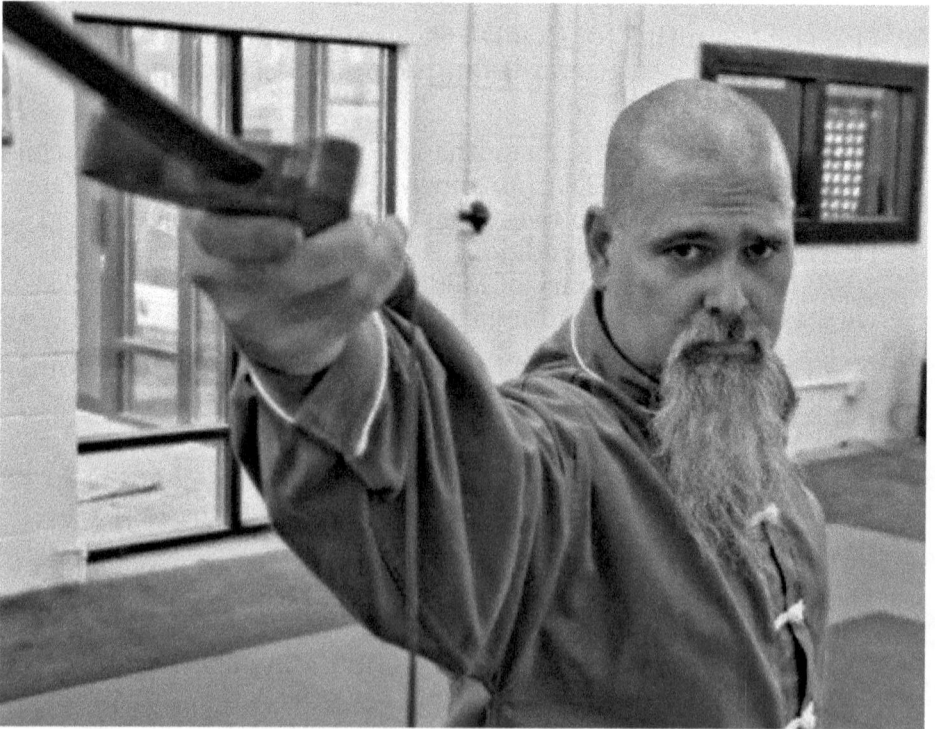

www.ingramcontent.com/pod-product-compliance
Lightning Source LLC
Chambersburg PA
CBHW062133040426
42335CB00039B/2097